Is your brain making you fat?

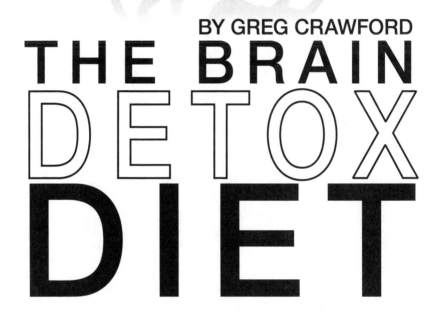

BY GREG CRAWFORD

THE BRAIN
DETOX
DIET

"How to tap into your inner strength and focus to create a new and leaner body"

ISBN: 0989022714
ISBN 13: 9780989022712

Library of Congress Control Number: 2014936721
It's a Lifestyle Fitness, Morristown, NJ

CONTENTS

ACKNOWLEDGMENT

Dedicated to my parents: my mother Nancy for always supporting me no matter what and my father Wayne who is reading this book in heaven and proud.

The people in your life that you impact in a positive way, whether few or many, is what's important. Also, what your purpose is and who you are is what defines you. During those times of darkness, it is with a clear purpose, faith and perseverance that the light will shine brighter than ever.

INTRO

Great job getting this book! Everything I'm going to teach in this book has been a game changer for me in my life. All of these tools have not only allowed me to look and feel great physically, but my laser sharp focus allows me to achieve goal after goal. I feel unstoppable by following the brain detox properties!

We live in a toxic world right now surrounded by things that are toxic to our minds and toxic to our bodies. If you want to become a motivated, laser sharp focused, LEAN machine, then follow this plan I have outlined for you NOW. I developed this idea, or what I would like to call a *movement*, to give you the tools you need to detox the brain as well as the body. I believe in helping you to be your best from the inside out. Everything is connected. Often life and healthy habits work parallel with each other. The health of your body can be a direct reflection of what's in your mind. If we can improve your thoughts and feelings, then I believe the body will follow.

Disclaimer: I am not a psychiatrist or a doctor. I am a fitness entrepreneur. I am a constant student of personal growth, nutrition and attend seminars to listen to the world's greatest and most successful motivational speakers and self help authors. I have also spent years working with hundreds of people and clients to help motivate them to lose weight or simply look and feel their best. I am looking forward to share my knowledge and experience with you.

What does personal growth mean to you? For me, it's a never-ending journey to evolve, find balance, increase wisdom and knowledge, love deeper and contribute more. We are all a work in progress. I have not met anyone as of yet who is perfect and has it all completely worked out. If you are not constantly growing as a person, then you are seriously under utilizing your gift. That gift is not a talent that you possess or singular character strength. That gift is to be the best version of YOU for the world. Growth is not meant to be done alone. As humans we were built to thrive off each other as a community. True growth starts with the help of others... Others you **trust**. Whether they are friends, family, coworkers, gym buddies, personal trainers or life coaches. Growth is only possible with the strength of your support system or like-minded individuals in your life. I don't know about you, but trust is not something that comes easy for me. How many times have you questioned the motives of someone who wants to help? Many times I've sought out advice and friendships, yet was unable to grow from the experience due to my lack of trust in them.

So how do we trust? To me, trust starts with the truth. When I turn to someone I trust, I know that I will hear the truth. Whether I like it or not.

When I started my business a few years ago I joined a group of like-minded men who owned their own businesses and shared the same overall vision of life. I've been approached and have thought about joining other similar groups but always hesitated. There was something different about this group and the man that created it. The difference that pulled me in was that with these guys, no matter what, I got the truth. This was sometimes the hard truth. As one of my mentors, Paul Reddick, would often say, "All progress starts with the truth." So, in the beginning of the book, I will be sharing some of my hard truths with you and hope to be your trusted source to improve your life. I will help you along your journey into a more focused and forever lasting healthy lifestyle.

5 TELL TALE SIGNS YOU NEED A BRAIN DETOX IS IF YOU SUFFER FROM:

1. You are hyper-sensitive
2. You tend to make poor decisions
3. You engage in emotional eating
4. You feel burnt out
5. You lack focus and motivation

I know right off the bat you can pick out at least one or two of the above that are currently affecting you. I know I can. That's why it's going to be very important for you to absorb the advice I'm going to give you. The great thing about the Brain Detox is that you can continue to revisit the tools I will map out for you to keep yourself grounded on your future path. If you could tap into someone's mind and change their way of thinking, you have then established the groundwork to change their habits and ultimately change their body. It's not just by receiving the information. You have to begin by tapping into the subconscious mind, which is our programmed way of thinking that ultimately controls our actions. You are probably very in touch you're your conscience, the voice in your head that helps you make decisions between right and wrong. It tends to be the louder and more present voice that speaks to you in your head. However, your subconscious is layered with experiences and agreements you formed with yourself from your past that affects every decision you make along with your actions. Right now it may be automatic for you to turn to food when put in a situation where you're stressed or emotional. If you can improve your subconscious thinking, you'll improve the automatic action on how you make choices and live your life. Many fitness professionals and nutritionists don't think about that, they just give you the information and expect you to change. Think about how powerful your subconscious is. There might be events from your past as a young child that still effect how you react to certain situations. Maybe it was a parent who was afraid to let you take chances or take risks, so now you get stuck in your comfort zone.

Before you can commit to a serious diet, you first must detox the brain and follow the advice laid out for you. The hard truth is that no diet is going to work unless your brain is hardwired to be focused and clear on its goal. This is exactly what the brain detox is going to do for you: clear out the "noise" and get you programmed to make the right decisions in your life, especially when it comes to eating.

Before we begin, I'm going to tell you my story and how I got so involved with personal growth, fitness and nutrition. I experienced my own highs and lows in life. However, those experiences made me who I am today because I made the best of all my personal growth experiences. I have used the tools I learned in life to help other people get through difficult situations in their lives. Growing up I was a very good athlete. That was my identity. My love for athletics, working out and playing football was a big part of my life and was #1 on my priority list even before school. This identity would take me into college, where as a freshman I was still excelling in football.

However, by the beginning of my junior year of college, my path and identity would change. It was the very first game of the season and I was covering a wide receiver when I went to make a sharp cut and planted my foot in the dirt. My body was moving pretty fast in one direction but when my foot pushed off the ground I felt a pop and my knee slid out of its socket. I went down quickly. After the game I went for an MRI and the very next day got the news that I had torn my ACL ligament. If you don't know anything about ACL'S, it's a pretty important ligament that holds your knee together when playing sports like football. A blown ACL is a season ending injury. At this point I was overwhelmed with shock and a feeling of emptiness. Football had been such an instrumental part of my life for the past 9 years and was always my main focus. Now that's it! For the first time in my life I was not playing. I remember after my surgery I went to a game to cheer on my teammates and sat with some of the guys I was friendly with who didn't play but were just there to cheer and drink beer. I can remember feeling completely disconnected with not only the team, but also with playing the game altogether. It was a feeling I was not used to. After that, I never went back to watch nor be a part of the game of football. This was a decision I would later regret.

Over the next few months I had some complications with my knee and didn't have full range of motion. It was getting very frustrating and I was nervous that I would end up with a slight limp. I would eventually go in for another surgery that year and just found myself getting more depressed, while popping my pain pills like candy and sitting on the couch. I dropped all my classes, and the fall semester of my junior year turned out to be a wash.

After the last surgery I finally started to develop a greater range of motion in my knee and began feeling more confident to get up and do more. My roommate at the time was a former player from New Jersey and was into working out at the gym. He encouraged me to get off the couch and go to the gym with him and over time I started to feel like myself again. However, one apparent change was that I no longer had the responsibility of reporting to football practice and meetings, which had previously dominated my life. Now, with all this time on my hands, I became more enthralled with the gym and working out recreationally to enhance my physical appearance. The other new hobby I picked up was partying.

As we fast forward to my last semester of college, my plan was to go back home and join the FDNY while personal training on the side. However, the new identity that I formed after my football career came to an end would change all of that. From going out to clubs and bars, to hanging around the wrong people, I began doing things that were out of character for me. I started selling drugs. Ecstasy to be exact, a popular party drug in the 90's and early 2000's. Even though I battled my conscience knowing this was not the right way to start a business, I was a young kid who was enticed by the easy money and notoriety I was receiving.

Little did I know my plans would come to a screeching halt by the time I finished my last semester of school. My life was then forced to change course with an earth-shattering knock at my door. In an instance, my door was smashed open and I was being arrested. My heart sank in my chest and my body went numb. This had never been my long-term plan. I had only wanted to make enough money for myself without being too heavily involved. However, the damage had been done and it didn't even matter that I had been pulling myself away from this activity that I knew was wrong. I completely stopped selling ecstasy in my last semester of school based on the realization of what the repercussions were and how they could potentially affect my future. Following my arrest, I was released on bail and managed to finish school and return home to NY. You were probably thinking my time of darkness was when I got hurt and couldn't play football anymore. However, it was at this point in my life when the light began closing up on me, sending me into a peril of depression.

During the next three years while still out on bail and my case being postponed, I worked in a health club in NYC. This was the worst time of my life because even though I was out and working, I was looking at jail time for my prior actions. My depression prevented me from thriving at personal training because I didn't see any point in succeeding at anything. How can I be a positive, motivated coach for someone when I'm looking at jail time? As you can imagine, all I was doing was feeling sorry for myself; which today is one of my big no no's. While all my friends were getting good jobs and meeting their spouses, I could only think that I would be the loser who went to jail and couldn't get a job. I was supposed to do great things with my life, and there I was wasting my days waiting to go to prison and then be a bum. Yes, those were my thoughts and the demons were singing masterpieces in my head. I can even recall being out with my friends in Brooklyn one night. It felt like everything was in slow motion just watching all my best friends who were having such a good time and were so happy. I freaked out and left without saying anything. That night I was driving over the bridge to get home when I thought about suicide. I actually thought about smashing my car over the bridge. Obviously I didn't take action on that thought, but I was seriously contemplating this in my head! The point is, I didn't see any light at the end of the tunnel, until that one day came.

The day I was sentenced, the judge sentenced me to 2 and half years in federal prison. I would serve 2 of those years away in a prison in the middle of nowhere in Pennsylvania. I remember actually leaving the courtroom with a sense of relief, as though a huge weight had been lifted off my shoulders. All I had to do now was the time. Start the clock, please! During that time away, I was actually in a much better place mentally. There was light at the end of the tunnel now. I guess you can say I found myself and found appreciation for everything

I have. I spent most of that time in deep thought, reading and exercising. But what I also discovered was how reading books that were focused on making me a better person would change my life. I read one right after another and quickly realized how much I loved personal growth, success stories and motivation. Even though I was cutoff from the outside world, I felt at peace and a deeper connection with myself while reading greats like Tony Robbins, Napoleon Hill, Zig Ziglar, Jack Canfield and the list goes on. I educated myself on business, self-help, nutrition and psychology.

When I got out of jail, there was little opportunity for me with a felony record, and was lucky to have my cousin hire me to help run his construction business. It was an okay paying job at the time, but something inside me knew I was meant to do more by using my knowledge of fitness, nutrition and personal growth. **It was time to forge a new path**. I ended up leaving the construction business and took a job at a large health club as a personal trainer. Luckily, they liked my experience and the way I looked so I don't think they bothered with the background check. From there, I worked as a trainer but knew I still needed to do more to create something that truly helps people to reach for their best. It was time to start my own business. After one year I quit my job at the gym and went out on my own. I then set another goal where in the following year I would hire another trainer and begin building the business. After one year of renting space from a smaller private gym, I saved up a few bucks, got a loan, used a few credit cards and found a perfect starter space to open my own gym. This was just the beginning of my commitment towards helping people through fitness, nutrition and personal growth. From that gym I expanded into a larger facility and grew the business while reaching hundreds of people. This was the foundation.

After creating a popular and successful 30-day weight loss detox challenge, I started applying the Brain Detox principles with the people in my area, which helped them make lasting changes in their lives. From the request of many, I wrote this book to share with the world my principles and philosophies along with my own personal story. We all create our own prisons for ourselves, but with the right mindset and direction, you can break free from whatever is holding you back from being the healthy and happy person you know is there.

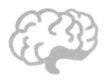

Chapter 1
HAVING A STRONG ENOUGH "WHY"

One of the biggest keys to having the motivation and focus to plow through any goal (especially weight loss) is doing everything with a higher purpose. You've probably heard remarkable stories of people, who under crazy extreme circumstances, had the will to live and survived a near death experience.

Did you hear the story of the hiker who fell into a canyon and got his arm trapped between two boulders? His story was made into a movie called 127 hours. For days he was trapped in isolation while he started growing weak and slowly dying. His desire to live was so great, that this man amputated his own arm with a pocketknife to free himself and find help. Now that's motivation and a strong "why"!

How about Viktor Frankl, the author of "Man's Search for Meaning"? Viktor was a prisoner in the concentration camps during WWII. He described how everyday, no matter how extreme the conditions were, he kept his mind and body moving forward because his life had such meaning. His "why" was that strong. While many lost hope, Viktor knew in his heart that love, courage and significance was such a deep part of him. Even under such harsh circumstances, he continued to live for that higher purpose.

Do you think if your life depended on it at this very moment, you would do what it takes to motivate yourself? Motivation doesn't exist because you don't need motivation. You need a strong enough "why" and to tap into your primitive instincts to fight for what you want without the option of quitting. It's as though your life depends on it! It's in your DNA to have the will of a lion and the fight of a Spartan warrior! What's it going to take for you to go inside and reach your deepest human trait to push you further? A near death experience?

You need to start with a support system and a strong enough "why". Superficial "whys" will never last. Everything has a deeper purpose.

Example: You want to lose weight and look good.

Superficial why: To look and feel good in a bathing suit.

Higher purpose "Why": I want to look my best so my future spouse sees how healthy I am on the outside to match the person on the inside. I also want to be a leader to my children and teach them by example how to take control of their lives and be healthy.

You are a real life hero. Your life is your story. So how will it be told? Every story has victims and every story has a hero. So who will you be: the victim or the hero? It doesn't matter where you are in your story. We are all at different places in our story. But I think there is a hero in all of us. You are a hero! You are NOT the victim. To be a hero is not always exciting. To be a hero means that there is some suffering. To be a hero means that there is no perfect timeline. But I guarantee you that YOU are a hero to someone or even many. It's time you realize this and answer the call. There are people out there who count on you! These can be people very close to you or people you haven't even touched yet. How you've lived and how you live from this day forward will determine who has found that hero in you. I have quite a few people in my life that are my heroes! If you can feel overwhelmed, cheated and full of fear, then that's the victim of the story talking. Which you are not! The hero carries the weight of the world. The hero doesn't let their past define them. The hero makes big decisions with faith close to heart and leads through their actions. The hero will win and lose battles and will have peaks and valleys. The hero will accept the losses and rise above the valleys, while enjoying the wins and souring high amongst the peaks. You are a hero to someone and at any point you can change your story and the direction you are heading. Keep creating that hero's story. That is your "why".

GREG'S PIA'S (Put Into Action)

- Have a clear vision of what exactly you want and how you want to look and feel.

- Ask yourself, "Why do I want that?" and "What will that ultimately do for me?"

- Ask, "Who am I a hero to and who will benefit from me being at your best?"

- Buy the outfit you want to look great in or create your vision board.

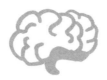

Chapter 2

YOUR ENERGY IS SACRED!

We all contain something special that we need in order to move through life with purpose. However, our supply is limited so keep it sacred so you can use it where needed most. What I'm talking about is our energy. You might also call this your power or aura. This is not the typical kind of energy that we get from food and need to run around all day. The type of energy I'm explaining to you is your energy field, your positive energy field to be exact.

If you broke down the human body under a microscope trillions of times, you would find that our bodies are made up of individual cells. Each individual cell is made up of particles, and these particles are constantly in motion. This constant movement is what forms our energy. If you really think about it on a deeper level, we're all made up of energy.

This is very powerful because as you know, there are positives and negatives jumping back and forth between this energy. I know you have probably heard of the law of attraction and "the secret." There is definitely validity to the law of attraction, but it goes way beyond just thinking a constant thought and attracting that. There's more to it. It's how you react to each situation that determines what you attract. That's the *real* secret.

Years ago there was this wacky looking guy with long hair who discovered "the real" weight loss solution. Most diet books and fitness entrepreneurs will tell you that you have to workout at least three times per week and eat a perfect diet or stick to certain foods in order to lose weight. You probably already know that, right? However, it does not always work that way. If it were that simple, you would not be struggling with your weight still. Don't get me wrong, those two things are very important. However, it's easier said than done. This man may not have looked like a diet and fitness professional, but he did discover something groundbreaking that effects you everyday and can be the deciding factor in whether you can overcome that annoying weight loss problem. His name was Albert Einstein. You're probably saying, "Greg, what does he have to do with weight loss?" Well, Albert Einstein developed the idea that all matter is the sum of moving particles and atoms, which equals energy. This energy is the key to your weight loss. Let me explain. If all matter is made of energy that would mean each individual body has its own energy field. There is a constant transferring of this energy going on around you. Some people and places give off a higher degree of positive energy than others.

How does this affect weight loss? If you plan on following through with a strict weight loss diet and workout regimen, you're going to need a constant flow of positive energy to keep you focused on that path. That constant flow of positive energy is what keeps your mindset in the state to lose the weight. Anyone can bombard you with diet information and grueling workouts, but it's your energy that keeps you focused on your goals.

My message to you is "keep your energy sacred" and get around the right people that will elevate you to new heights with your goals.

I want you to try something with me. Stand up. Open your hands, palms facing each other about 6 inches apart. What I'd like you to do for the next 30 seconds is move your hands back and forth in front of each other as fast as you can. Continue this action at this speed for 30 seconds while keeping the palms of your hands 6 inches apart. From there, you're going to stop, slow it down, and just rotate your hands in small circles with your palms facing each other. What do you feel between your hands? More than likely, as you move your hands slower you're going to feel the transfer of energy between the palms of your hands.

When you're interacting with other people there's energy being transferred. There can be positive energy, as well as negative energy being transferred. Always remember that your energy is sacred.

A great book I recommend to all my clients on how to keep your energy sacred is 'Silent Power' by Stewart Wilde. Stewart Wilde is an energy and spiritual guru. In 'Silent Power' he talks about how everyone has their own energy field and describes how people with positive energy have a more solid energy field. On the other hand, someone with a lot of negative energy contains a wild energy field resembling a web, with arms flaring out, attempting to pull at and absorb the positive energy of those around it.

He also discusses that it's important for you not to lean into someone's positive energy too much. If you're always leaning into someone else's positive energy, eventually, they're going to pull back because you're going to take away from the energy that they are harnessing. Try not to lean into positive people too much. Instead, surround yourself with positive like-minded people, while maintaining your own energy by protecting it and creating more vibration within yourself. Elevate yourself to a higher level. Have you ever been around certain people with such radiant energy and realize that you actually feel their energy? It lifts you up a little, right? That could happen anywhere. Conversely, you may also have found yourself in a room filled with negative energy wondering to yourself, "Why am I in here?" You can walk into virtually any room and be aware of the energy that is being emitted. However, it is only when you allow yourself to connect with that energy that a bond is formed or a boundary is placed.

Your energy is sacred. If you're giving it away to negativity or pulling from someone else's positive energy all the time, you're never going to live out your full potential, achieve greatness or enhance the lives of the people you love.

Sometimes you will face opposition from those people that don't understand where you're at or the direction you are headed in. You will be judged and people will always have their opinions about you. There will be people who will follow you to the ends of the earth and those who will question your every move. Whether they are friends, peers, customers, strangers or family members, the only person questioning you that you have to answer to is YOURSELF. You know in your heart when you are making the best decisions for YOU. No one else can decide what's best for you but YOU. For example, when it comes to changing your eating habits and living a healthy lifestyle friends may say you're fine the way you are or question why you are eating so healthy or why are you not drinking. Maybe it's your spouse that doesn't like change and is afraid how they will be affected by it. When you follow your heart knowing know that what you do is with all the best intentions then there is no reason to defend yourself. After all, if you try to defend your every move, you will only be left exhausted and frustrated. It's a losing battle to get everyone on board at all times. What matters is that you are on board with your own decisions at all times. Only you live your life. Only you fight your fights. Only you believe in your visions. Change because you want to change. Be confident in your decisions. Be yourself and be fearless about it.

A good friend once told to me that I was losing my edge during a time when I was trying to grow my business. At the time, I was putting a lot of my energy into a relationship that was consuming it all and it began affecting other areas of my life especially work. Because I was not protecting and maintaining my own energy, I constantly felt drained and was not able to give my energy to areas of my life that really demanded my attention. "Keep your energy sacred" is something I have said to many clients recently and has become a key factor in what I believe allows us to lead a life of happiness and focus. We only have a certain amount of energy. Protect it.

The trick is not giving your energy away all the time so that you may use it when needed to improve your life. The people you love most in your life will benefit more from you when you keep your positive energy sacred.

Each and every day we are faced with challenges that may leave us feeling upset, frustrated or even offended by the words and actions of those around us. Maybe the day's plans didn't work out, or somebody was rude at the office, or a job that should have taken one hour took three. It could be the number you see on the scale, or that the stock market is down, that your child didn't make a team, or maybe you wish you had a nicer boss. Maybe it's on a more personal scale where your spouse is making you unhappy. Life is full of challenges and disappointments. There will always be interruptions and difficulties. We cannot control every circumstance. However, we can control our reactions, choices and actions moving forward. Too many people have the wrong approach to life. They think they can't be happy unless they avoid disappointment and have complete control over everything in their lives. That is not realistic. You have to believe or trust that if your plans don't work out, you will still be able to find happiness. Everybody doesn't have to treat you right for life to be enjoyable. No matter what happens, you can find peace, enjoy the day, and at the very least, pray for those who upset you. They need it more than you! Life is too short to be upset and offended. If you allow other people to control your joy, there will always be some reason to be discouraged. Remember, every time you do this you are giving away your energy. When you protect and keep your energy sacred, you truly take control of yourself and make choices with a better frame of mind, body, and spirit. All we have to do is use the energy we have and rise above it all.

THE WEIGHT OF THE WORLD

Sometimes we feel like we're carrying the weight of the world on our shoulders. Have you ever felt that way? You don't have to carry it alone. I heard a wise man tell another man, "Life is too short to put your energy into things or people that weigh you down." Remove some of that weight from your shoulders and lighten the load. Life is too short! We say it all the time, but it's a powerful statement. It's time to conduct a WEIGHT OF THE WORLD audit.

The following are some examples of the weight you might be carrying around. From the following list, which can you start systematically distancing from or removing from your life?

- Negative people
- Gossip
- Doom and gloom of "the news"
- Debt
- Toxic food
- Abusive people
- People that are takers only
- Trying to "fit in" all the time

- Hiding from truth
- Re-living the past instead of living today
- Trying to be perfect
- Dwelling on your current circumstances instead of either changing it or embracing it

This is your life to live. Nobody else is living your life. Forge your own path with less weight and see how much further you can go! Life is as good as you make it. Not everyday is going to "rock" all the time. You're not always going to kick butt and sometimes life just kicks your butt. That's reality, but it's ok! Just because you have a bad day or two or even three, does not mean you should get discouraged and lose track of your goals. That's a whole part of the journey, my friends. We are supposed to face obstacles and catch a blow to the ego once in a while. A part of life is getting tested. The universe does a perfect job of testing us from our faith to our strength right down to our soul. How you react to these tests will determine your success. You can either throw your hands up in the air declaring to all of Facebook and your peers that you give up, or you can embrace life's tests and slowly work through each challenge. When you do this you will learn more about yourself and become a stronger, smarter, more resilient person, especially when you overcome each challenge with integrity. Just keep in mind that amongst the chaos comes change and this will only bring you closer to your goals and dreams.

Have you ever been on a boat out at sea? Have you ever gotten seasick? What's the first thing they tell you? Keep your eyes on the horizon. Life is like the sea. It's going to knock you around and the water will sometimes get very rough. With the turmoil of the rough seas (which can make you sick to your stomach at times), raise your chin and keep your eyes on that horizon! The horizon is where your goals lie. Don't get caught up in the rockiness around you. Keep your focus on the stillness of the horizon and you won't feel sick. Remember, how you react to situations will determine what you attract. That's the key to keeping your energy sacred.

"KEEP YOUR EYES ON THE HORIZON"

GREG'S PIA'S (Put Into Action)

- Begin saying no to things or people that suck your energy.

- Start setting boundaries around people in your life that you care about but are dragging you down.

- Immediately remove yourself from negative situations.

- Start surrounding yourself with more like-minded people who share your goals.

- Set daily positive reminders in your phone.

- When life throws you a curveball, remember to stay focused on your horizon. The curveball is temporary and every problem has a solution.

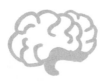

Chapter 3
YOUR BRAIN POWER

You have something very powerful inside you: the power of your brain. This power we possess in our brains can either work greatly for you or against you. Everything that the human race has created was discovered by our use of brainpower. Our brains control everything we do and we move in the direction to which we are programed. So if our brains are not programmed to eat healthy and make good choices, then no matter how hard we consciously try to use our will power, the power of the subconscious will take over. Our subconscious mind determines most of our conscious decision-making.

You may have tried different diets and programs to lose weight in the past. Maybe you have tried to stay motivated and focused only to fall back into old habits without making any true breakthroughs. Wondering why you can't stay motivated and focused for the long haul, or lose weight and keep the weight off for the long haul? It all starts with the brain. In the following chapters, I'm going to break that down for you and give you a game plan to re-program your brain to start making all the right choices along with a stress free approach to eating right.

Let's break down your brainpower into two parts: the conscious mind and the unconscious mind. Your conscious mind makes up about 10% of your total brainpower, and your subconscious makes up 90% of your total brainpower. That's a lot of power behind your thoughts and actions.

What your conscious mind controls is your front-of-mind awareness. It controls your short-term memory, and controls your willpower. Your subconscious, which is 90% of your brainpower, (and it's better known as your primal brain) controls your emotions and feelings, your creativity, your habits, your focus and your long-term memory. Subconscious is defined as anything in the mind that cannot be consciously processed in the moment but can be recalled.

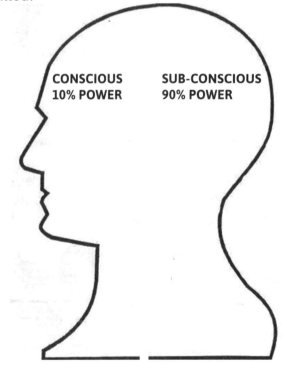

CONSCIOUS
10% POWER

SUB-CONSCIOUS
90% POWER

YOUR CONSCIOUS MIND CONTROLS:

- Front of mind awareness
- Short term memory
- Will power

YOUR SUBCONSCIOUS MIND CONTROLS:

- Emotions and feelings
- Creativity
- Habits
- Focus
- Long-term memory

Most of the important decisions you make come from your emotions and feelings or your habits. Have you ever gone to purchase a new car with a game plan of getting the best deal, but than you "fall in love" with a certain car and end up making a purchase based on emotions? That was a subconscious decision. You might be happy with the deal you got, but it's more than likely that you also went a little above and beyond with your finances to get the car you wanted. Typically, when you go on a diet plan, you're trying to use your conscious mind to make these decisions on what to eat, and what not to eat every day. We start to use our willpower to consciously alter or change our sub-conscious habits. As you know, wills were meant to be broken. You're really only tapping into 10% of your brainpower to keep yourself motivated and focused. Eventually the overpowering subconscious takes over. If you truly want long term and automatic success, it all starts in the subconscious. It is important to focus on and be mindful of is what's going on in the subconscious and what you're allowing in that part of your mind. We live in a toxic world, whether it's the food we eat, the environment, the air that we breathe, or sometimes the people that we're around. A lot of different things affect your brain and your subconscious mind that you're not even aware of. In turn, that effects your conscious decision-making, which has likely been the cause of why your diets have failed in the past and have left you unfocused and unmotivated.

You've got to start changing the thought patterns in your head. Thought patterns that have been put in your head by your parents, teachers, your mentors growing up, and the circumstances that you were exposed to are the thoughts you must pay careful attention to. Those are the thought patterns that have an effect on how you feel about yourself. Odds are you're probably sabotaging yourself, not from the knowledge or the information out there, but from your own head. All of us have a movie playing in our heads from our past, present and it even projects what our future looks like. Imagine a rerun of this movie playing in your head over and over again. Your subconscious plays a major role in what this movie looks like. Your subconscious mind will actually affect what you do in the outside world. When you're listening to talk radio, or the news, reading or listening to gossip, with nothing but negativity impacting you, what do you think will be the theme of the movie playing in your head? Is it positive or is it negative? Your actions will tell the answer because they follow the thoughts that occupy your mind.

Many times we let our emotions get the best of us and we often turn to food to make us feel better in stressful situations. Emotional eating can be considered one of the leading causes for weight gain. Don't fool yourself into thinking that you are stronger than your emotions. Instead take a different approach...Improve your emotions. And remember that negative emotions are temporary.

In my program, the Brain Detox Diet Program, we're going to start with the brain portion of the detox because that's going to be the most important part. It is only then that we can discuss nutritional science. We first need to focus on detoxing the brain, most importantly the sub-conscious part of the brain. I'm going to tell you exactly how to do that. It's going to get you super- charged and fired-up. You're going to wake up every day motivated, focused, and confident in your ability to make good decisions in your eating and in your life automatically. After that, we will look at more specific ways of eating stress which will help you achieve weight loss and a strong, healthy body. By then, you're going to become a new energized person who is ready begin forging a new path of success.

How do we tap into our primal inner focus and motivation? We have to improve the sub-conscious. It starts by eliminating or setting boundaries with the "noise" in our heads. The next chapter will be dedicated to identifying the "noises" and where they come from. After identifying the "noises" we're going to replace them with my six key motivators in chapter 6. Pay very close attention and follow my plan of cleaning up your sub-conscious brain because in the end I promise you that you will begin to see lasting results. I've experienced the results first hand along with a countless number of clients that I've worked closely with in the past.

GREG'S PIA'S (Put Into Action)

- Realize that your subconscious controls your actions.

- Protect your subconscious mind and what you allow to enter it.

- You can change the patterns of your subconscious with the Brain Detox tools.

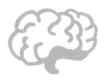

Chapter 4

ELIMINATING OR SET BOUNDARIES WITH THE 5 "NOISES" IN OUR SUB-CONSCIOUS MIND

The 5 "noises" are made up of the following:

- Negativity
- Fear
- Distrust
- Anger
- Worry

Do you disguise most emotions as stress? All of the emotions listed above make up the "noise" that will eventually lead to STRESS. The noise that is hibernating within our subconscious minds is delivered to us through messages. We can find these mediums that deliver the messages from a number of sources. You have to protect your mind and decide which thoughts are important to entertain and which are not. It's not your job to listen to and absorb all the noise. Your job is to make room and be clear to make smart decisions to better your life. Everyday we're bombarded with messages of negativity, fear, dis-trust, anger and worry. These messages can be received subconsciously through people we surround ourselves with, specifically people who tend to carry negativity. We also get these messages from TV, specifically the news and reality TV. Even when it comes to politics and religion we are often getting messages of worry, distrust, anger and fear. I'm not saying all TV is bad, all people are bad or all politics and religion are bad. What I'm saying is that we need to start being more mindful of the effects that result from getting caught up in the parts of these things that create those "noises". There is much we can avoid and our children can avoid to prevent the negative messages from entering. This will create more room for a more positive environment in our own head. **This is the key to long-term success**.

Let me give you an example of just how powerful messages to our subconscious are, good or bad. Finish this sentence: "The best part of waking up"...

Did you say, "Is Folgers in the cup"? I'm assuming most of you reading this book remember the commercial for Folgers coffee. That tagline is a message we received quite often watching that commercial. Now I'm not sure how many times you may have seen that, but imagine receiving messages daily that have projected "noise" related feelings. It's a safe bet that you're storing those feelings subconsciously and carrying them with you. Let's take a closer look at our emotions that make up the "noise" in our heads to have a better awareness on how to deal with them better.

NEGATIVITY

Do you surround yourself with people that carry negative energy? The energy that you're getting from some people could be toxic to you. Not all people with negative energy are bad people, however, their energy can still be toxic to you. So, you can either remove them from your life or set boundaries. Always do your best to protect the positive flow of energy in your life by avoiding the negativity of those around you. You should not allow someone else's negativity to get in the way of how you're feeling or how you want to live. Don't get caught up in other people's "stuff". Gossip is only wasted energy.

Practice the art of not giving your negative thoughts power. Every time you say or write a negative thought about yourself, you give it power. Let's be very mindful of this and change the communication you have with yourself. What you say and write enters the universe will inevitably make up your reality.

Ex: I'm depressed, I can't do this, I wish I was in better shape, I'm lonely.

The law of attraction will work to keep you there. Remember, how you react to situations is what you will attract. Instead stop yourself from proclaiming that and change those words like: I want to feel better tomorrow.

I know I can do this over time. I'm looking forward to being in better shape and I want someone good to enter my life since they will see the best version of me now. We all have negative thoughts at times. However, it's the way we communicate them that we need to be mindful of. If you can control the communication of your thoughts, you will be able to make better choices and change your actions.

FEAR

Fear can be defined as False Evidence Appearing Real. Watching the news everyday or at night, you will find an underlining message of fear entering your sub-conscious. The news will project some really interesting stories and good news at times, but unfortunately most of what the media projects is bad news. So what is it that you are telling your subconscious mind? When you go to make a conscious decision the fear you absorbed in your subconscious mind is going to affect how you make that decision. When your mind is polluted with fear, it's hard to stay positive. Sometimes things happen that can make you question humanity, God, and all that is good especially when it comes to tragedy. You can question why things happen in the world, question your government and politicians, question why murderers and terrorists exist, or question God as to why there is such evil in the world. But dwelling on such negative thoughts will do you and the world no good. Right now it is important to focus on what is happening in your world. Place your focus not on the questions you have with the world around you but on what you can influence for the future right now in your local community and not from the news on TV. As decades pass, we are bombarded with an increasing amount of toxic, influences from processed foods and chemicals to the media exploiting violence on TV and in video games. Most of these toxic influences have led us to sedentary lifestyles and all of these influences affect our mindset and decision-making. My message to you is this... turn off the news, take a break from all news, go move your body by taking a long walk or work out a little harder today and set a positive example for the next generation. Focusing only on what and whom you can influence will keep you in a positive mindset and away from fear. Start doubting your fears instead of yourself. Your answers are there no matter what. Fear is holding you back. Look within yourself and you'll find the answers.

DISTRUST

I'll admit that I have a tough time trusting. This is because this is probably the most common message we get throughout our lives. Many of us have been let down by people close to us or let down by an organization we've trusted. Almost daily we receive messages of distrust from things we hear, political differences, unfaithfulness, news of tainted foods we eat and sometimes people we cross paths with. All of these things throughout our lives have put our guards up. If you keep getting yourself caught up in these messages and reacting from past experiences, you are putting yourself at risk of not being open to wonderful people in your life and holding healthy relationships. The quicker you move away and set boundaries from messages of distrust, the quicker you will attract just the opposite.

WORRY

We all have worry, but we can't let it overtake us. We have to move away from it as much as possible or it will overtake our lives. For the most part I keep myself focused and pretty calm. But I am human and do worry about a lot of things. I worry about my family and any issues that arise. I worry about the gym that I own. I worry about helping and delivering results to my clients and all of my members. I worry about my employees, that they are making a good living. I worry about my members and their families and that everyone is healthy and happy.

But I'm not writing today about those worries. Do you want to know what my big worry is? I'm going tell you in a minute. The other day I was having a down day. I don't like days like this because I don't usually have them. But it's ok because we are all going to go through peaks and valleys. Then I thought to myself... I don't want to waste this day just being down on myself and stressed. So my big worry is this... Wasting another day! There are 365 days a year and life is short, so the days we have are limited in the grand scheme of things. Each day we have is a gift, and we should not waste even one. Now I understand some days are going to be better and more productive than others. However, my advice to you would be this: when you're having a bit of a down day, worrying or feeling unproductive, first move and push your body physically. Even if you don't feel up to it. Next, do just one productive thing to move you even just a little further. This can be something very small. The other day when I was feeling down, I drove myself to the park and ran. Then I continued to walk to clear my head. I felt much better afterwards and was thinking more clearly. When I got home, I got on the computer and did one little task to move a project I have been working on but lost some steam. I can't over emphasize the power of going for a long walk. It's like taking a mini-mind vacation from everything. When I was away for those two years in Federal prison, the one time I could be alone in my thoughts was when I went outside to the rec yard and walked around the softball field. It gave me piece of mind, great ideas and helped me escape for a minute. Are you going to worry? Probably, yes. But make every day count and keep moving forward! Oh, and kick major butt on the days you're feeling good!

ANGER

I think out of all the noises in our heads, anger is the least dangerous to us and actually sometimes needed. The issue is when and how we use it. Anger should only be used for two main reasons: to fight in order to physically protect yourself, or for passion and fuel to accomplish something that the naysayers or haters said you couldn't. That can then be used as your fuel for the fire. Instead of having a negative reaction to the anger, we can actually use it to our advantage and move ourselves further in life with it.

I don't know about you, but have you have ever been wronged by someone you trusted? Or maybe there are people that didn't believe in you and doubted you. Then there are the haters. These are the people who always hate on you because they have their own issues and insecurities.

You're reaction to the anger felt and how you use it will determine whether your life goes in a positive direction or negative one.

You can decide right now how to use your anger: you can try to push it to the side and forget, (even though it's almost impossible to,) and let it become negative and self-sabotaging, or use it as the fuel to ignite a fire within you. You can burn down debilitating bridges of the past that are holding you back from reaching your full potential.

It's time to channel that anger into a burning desire that can conquer any obstacle or goal! It can be fitness related, career, or life.

You don't think I'm going to make it? I'll show you! I'm just the fat kid? I'm going to push out a few more reps just when I think I'm done. Look at me now! You think I'm too old? I'll put my age to the test and show you I can accomplish anything at any age!

If any of this resonates with you, use it towards your advantage and take yourself further in life with that fire inside. Don't let it become a negative and debilitating feeling. Use the anger you feel to your advantage and allow it to push yourself further. Do this to the point where you can actually be thankful for the people that have angered you in the past. They are the ones that help ignite the fire that rages greatness inside of you.

You have to encounter as much negative feedback as positive feedback and reinforcement. Change the pattern, but also re-feed it. You have to empty out the toxic things and re-feed it with positive things; it gets filled up with a lot of negativity and a lot of "noise" which you have to empty out. You have to do it on a regular basis.

Removing the "noise" is only the first step. The second step will be replacing it. If you don't replace it with something else, the "noise" will always return quickly. The next chapter focuses on what to replace the "noises" with so you can go on and live your dreams as a focused, motivated, lean bodied machine.

GREG'S PIA'S (Put Into Action)

- Have more awareness where different negative messages come from and remove yourself from them.

- Be more selective of the TV that you and your children watch.

- Refrain from watching the news. If it's that important you will hear about it. You can be educated on the world without watching the news. Remember the media controls what they want you to see and hear.

- Change your communication. Remind yourself to speak and react differently. Your communication to the universe will attract what you reflect out. You are a reflection of your communication to the world.

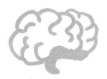

Chapter 5

REPLACE "THE NOISE" WITH THE 6 KEY MOTIVATORS

1. BREATHING
2. SLEEPING
3. MOVING
4. READING
5. ESCAPING
6. BELIEVING

In the previous chapter I talked about removing or setting boundaries with the "noise". Unless we replace it with something, that "noise" will always find its way back into our heads. This is why we replace them with the six Key Motivators. The six key motivators is a list of actions that we many times seem to neglect but are crucial for the health of the body and mind. Why, if they are so crucial, are they neglected? I think we know the benefits of each Key Motivator, however I don't think often we place them in the correct order of importance in our life. Just like I became aware of the messages I was receiving that created the "noise" in my head, it became aware to me over the course of my life experiences that all six Key Motivators tremendously helped me block out that "noise" and create a more focused and clear mind. This is exactly what I want to help you with.

BREATHING

A lot of times we forget to breathe. How many times has your mind been racing, and all of a sudden when you take a deep breath, it catches up to you. This is because you're not breathing correctly; you're taking shallow breath instead of taking slower deep breaths. You're holding your breath unconsciously. Shallow breathing limits the diaphragm from expanding and the amount of oxygenated air that you take in. According to Harvard Medical, people with chronic high blood pressure can lower it just by incorporating breathing exercises and techniques. Most people have developed poor breathing habits, thus further restricting oxygen intake. The resulting oxygen deficiency is having a negative effect on our health and our overall performance. Oxygen deprivation can be associated with all kinds of chronic diseases.

Breathing can be both conscious and unconscious. The respiratory center of the brain controls a person's normal breathing rate. A normal breathing pattern is automatic so you don't have to consciously think about it. Both voluntary breathing and automatic breathing both serve the purpose of getting oxygen into the bloodstream. Oxygen's main role in the blood stream is to transport oxygen into your cells. Our cells utilize this oxygen to produce ATP through a complex reaction called Cellular Respiration. ATP is your body's energy. Oxygen is also important for many other functions such as cellular repair and other biological reactions. So as you can see, without it we cannot sustain life. Knowing this importance should give us a better understanding of why we should put more emphasis on our breathing and begin to incorporate more breathing exercises into our daily routines.

Most diseases will not thrive in an oxygen-rich environment, according to Dr. James Balch, the author of The Super Antioxidants. If there is enough oxygen in our cells, degenerative disease cannot exist and metabolism functions more normally.

You can do voluntary deep breathing in many different forms: meditation, yoga, reflection, physical activity, or just breathing exercises. According to an article published by Sovik in 2000 on WebMD, there is a direct connection between the "prana" (or energy of breathing) and its effect on the body. This was observed in yoga and meditative exercises. Cellular metabolism, which is reactions in the cell to produce energy, is regulated by oxygen provided during breathing. The deep meditative breathing has been shown to positively affect immune function, hypertension, asthma, autonomic nervous system imbalance and stress related disorders.

One helpful exercise to do when you wake up in the morning before your kids get up is stand up, palms open, chest out, close your eyes and just focus on your breathing. This stance alone means a lot; you're opening yourself up. All day we are usually at the desk or in the car and we're closed up. Open yourself up for the day: it increases your natural, good hormones by doing this. Optimal breathing and integrating this awareness into your daily schedule is a must for optimal living and functioning. Once you get this right, you will begin to bring awareness to the difference between smooth, even breathing compared to sometimes erratic breathing.

SLEEPING

Every decade that goes by we become a more sleep-deprived society. The average sleep has decreased about two hours a night over the last thirty to forty years. It is said that now the average person sleeps six hours a night. I know people are different and some can function on less sleep than others, but the research is showing us just what lack of sleep is doing to us. According to an article in the Sleep Foundation, Kristen L. Knutson, PhD, Department of Health Studies, University of Chicago says, "There is laboratory evidence that short sleep durations of 4-5 hours have negative physiological and neurobehavioral consequences."

Three main benefits of getting close to eight hours of sleep include: your brain recharges, the cells in your body repair better, and you release the "good" hormones while sleeping. Did you know that you could die of sleep deprivation before dying of starvation? It's true. That's just how serious sleep is and yet we often neglect it. There are some other fun facts that I found out when researching the benefits of sleep. Did you know koala bears sleep the most at 22 hours a day and giraffes sleep the least on average 1.9 hours per day at 5-10 minute clips? A 2010 study found that C-reactive protein, which is associated with heart attack risk, was higher in people who got six or fewer hours of sleep a night. Sleep also improves physical performance. A Stanford University study found that college football players who tried to sleep at least 10 hours a night for seven to eight weeks improved their average sprint time and had less daytime fatigue and more stamina.

Researchers at the University of Chicago found that dieters who were well rested lost more fat -- 56 percent of their weight loss -- than those who were sleep deprived, who lost more muscle mass. Dieters in the study also felt hungrier when they got less sleep. "Sleep and metabolism are controlled by the same sectors of the brain," Dr. Rapoport says. "When you are sleepy, certain hormones go up in your blood, and those same hormones drive appetite."

There are other studies, which show that lack of sleep causes us to age more rapidly. That ties into the concept of cell repair and release of hormones, like growth hormones, while we sleep. Finally, as I discussed in previous chapters, the power of the subconscious, enables you to make better conscious decisions with the improvement of sleep. This allows you to lose weight much faster and easier than before.

Here are my quick tips to getting a good night sleep and extending it up to eight hours a night:

- Follow the Brain Detox properties (This alone will put your mind at rest)

- Re-train your internal clock by shutting off the TV and setting an earlier bedtime.
- Set your alarm clock to wake up one hour earlier than usual.
- Supplement with a Magnesium and Zinc capsule right before bedtime.
- Do some of the breathing or reading exercises at night

MOVING

We live in such a sedentary world. We're always in our cars, sitting at our desks and sitting on the couch. One of the most primitive and necessary features of being alive is movement. Our survival is reliant on moving our body. By moving I don't just mean walking from one seated area to the next. For moving to be considered a key motivator, it requires some form of strain on the body. This is in the form of exercise, running, hiking, biking, playing, fighting and lifting.

It's funny that movement is such a primitive basic and necessary feature; however many of us tell ourselves that we don't have time to do this. That way of thinking has got to change. It's probably the most important of all my key motivators because the benefits greatly out way that of any other motivating factor. And it is key to improving yourself. Also, when I talk about moving the body, I mean daily. We should be moving everyday. We spend such a great deal of time not moving that we must get some form of movement from what I previously mentioned in on a daily basis. Yes, your body was originally built to handle it. You just have to re-train it to do so.

Most of us know the benefits of moving the body and exercise, but let's go over some specifics. One of the biggest benefits is hormonal balance. I'm going to dive into some specifics about your hormones in a later chapter, but rigorous exercise is shown to increase the release of your good hormones, or hormones that offset the bad ones, like cortisol. Those bad hormones will wreak havoc on the body and emotional health. Also, many studies are showing the correlation between movement and exercise and how it boosts brain function. The results have been staggering, showing that as you increase movement, you increase overall brain function.

Another benefit is the metabolism of fat. When you move the body on a daily basis, your body becomes a well-oiled, functioning machine. Keep the machine going, otherwise if you turn it off for a while it becomes harder and harder to start back up. This goes much deeper than just calorie counting. I dislike calorie counting a great deal. If you're moving your body daily and adding bouts of higher intensity rigorous exercise with a clean, correctly proportioned diet full of antioxidant supplements, than you will be a healthy lean machine.

It's all about creating a more friendly balanced environment for your hormones, neurotransmitters, vitamins and minerals. Our bodies are a living miracle; just allow it to function properly by giving it what it needs.

READING

Growing up I hated to read. I'm sure if you have kids most of them do not have reading on their list of favorite things to do. As a matter of fact, even through college I somehow managed to get through school without reading a whole lot. I would call it more "scanning through textbooks." Unfortunately, or maybe I can say fortunately, the first book I read cover to cover that I actually enjoyed was when I went away to prison. It is unfortunate that I had to wait to go to prison to actually sit down and spend a little time to read a whole book. Being away from home and society got me to free up my mind and get dialed in with a lot of reading. Besides not having much else to do and the desire to keep out of trouble, I wanted to spend that time I had as productive as possible. So I read whatever I can get my hands on that had anything to do with improving myself. I wanted to improve my mindset, my body and my spirit and that's exactly what reading did for me. Now I know most who are reading this are not in prison, hopefully. My point is that reading books dramatically increased my motivation and focus. There is so much out there that we can learn from brilliant minds and topics to move us further in life. As we speak you are reading this book, which has a purpose of moving you further in your life. From books alone, I educated myself in holistic nutrition, which during my prison time worked towards a master's degree. I also studied the best of the best in personal growth, self-help and psychology. Today when I meet or speak with coaching clients, one of their homework assignments is to read a book each month that will inspire them to move forward in life and improve their well being. When you're reading, you're accepting messages into your brain, which feeds you trust, love, and all these good feelings.

ESCAPING

Escaping can happen in a variety of ways: vacations, breaks and pulling back a little or going to motivational events. These escapes can be daily, weekends or even longer. You need to feel an increase of energy from nature and groups of positive people. Not too long ago I was standing in a room in front of my peers. Normally I'm considered a pretty creative and focused guy in that particular group. However, that day I had a look on my face that said, "I'm burnt out". Do you know that look or feeling? Leading up to this day I took on a pretty big project, which was the expansion of my gym. It was a BIG project and a bit stressful. However, with some time and the help of a great team, things got done and now I can say things are flowing nicely. Let's go back to that look on my face...

While standing there in front of the group, the best advice I ever got was...TAKE A BREAK. Sounds so simple, but when you're always on overdrive, your brain starts to get cluttered and break down. That can kill your creativity, focus and motivation. So, I did just that and left my normal environment for a little bit... and boom! The creative juices started flowing again! This is just a spoke on the wheel of things you might need to do to detox your brain when feeling unmotivated, unfocused and unproductive. During this time, I had an epiphany and discovered quite a few other tools needed in a brain detox that keeps you highly focused, motivated and simply ready to conquer life.

Today is your escape day. Reading this book is your escape. Today is the day you officially step into the next stage of your life. Today is the day you escape from poor health or that feeling of not being at your best and not liking what you see in the mirror. I don't know where you are. I don't know why you are reading this book. Maybe you are at the perfect place in your life. Maybe you have a body that doesn't quit. Maybe you are at your best for your family.

Then again, maybe you want to take action to manifest a body of your dreams that will enable you to do all the activities you want. You want to wake up and feel energized. You want to be the most positive, motivated and focused you. This is the place you can finally be FREE.

BELIEVING

We are owned by our belief systems. Leave your old belief systems behind. When you do this, negative self-talk will kick in. Suspend all beliefs and just go for it. Practice visualization. It's okay to fall off course sometimes; it happens to us all. What's important is that you have the right path forged for yourself and you know where you're going. Know that wherever you are in life, you have the power and guidance to forge a new path for yourself if your current path does not serve you. Do you see where your path is leading you? Not sure? Then answer this: Is it in the direction that serves your core values in life? If not, then redirect and get back on course. Remember, you can only be guided if you know where you want to be.

The definition of perseverance is to persist in anything undertaken, while maintaining a purpose in spite of difficulty, obstacles or discouragement. The opposite of persevere would be to give up and quit. We've all been affected in one way or another by adversity in our life and have persevered through it. Why? Because we have to. We were built for it. Don't expect someone else to magically change your current situation or circumstances. You can! You are going to improve your own situation, improve your own health care, and help make this world a better place. You are going to persevere through any situation, circumstance or obstacle. But, you're not going to wait for something bad to happen with your health to begin this journey.

Persevere with everything you do! Take each day on with perseverance, persist in everything undertaken, and maintain a purpose in spite of difficulty, obstacles or discouragement. You can change your own circumstances because you have the power to do that now and everyday.

I believe that faith is something that is very personal. Yes, there are times when our faith is tested. I know that first hand; however, our faith and prayers are special gifts we are given, and believing that there is something bigger than us and our prayers are answered is a very deep feeling that you must have. Sometimes our prayers are answered and sometimes that higher being may say no. But he always is there for you, even on those bad days.

What do believe in? God, Jesus, Allah, Mohammad, evolution, yourself, ancient aliens, Buddha, spirits, the universe? Whatever you believe in you are supposed to have faith in. This is the faith that in the end everything is going to work itself out. But how much faith do you have when life throws you a curve ball or kicks you when you're down? It's easy to believe when things are going well and you feel great like nothing can stop you. But how's your faith when your back is up against the wall with the weight of the world is on your shoulders, and when things seem so bleak. Are you going to pack it in? Are you going to let your internal demons win and live in fear? You can't have faith unless it's tested. Without putting you to the test, faith is just another 5-letter word. You cannot possibly believe in something unless your faith is tested. So the next time you feel like, "I can't accomplish this," you believe even harder and show whatever higher power you believe in, that your faith is unbreakable.

GREG'S PIA'S (PUT INTO ACTION)

- Spend a few minutes early in the morning or in the evening before bed to focus on breathing. Listen to a meditation audio or just pay attention to your breathing and clear the mind.

- If you practice the Brain Detox properties, your sleep should improve. Set your alarm an hour earlier and get to bed an hour earlier. Change your sleep clock during the week.

- Set a consistent gym schedule. If you're not at the gym, go on long walks outside. If you're at the office, put in a solid fifty minute work session and then take a break to walk around.

- Make it a point to read thirty minutes a day. Pick books that will inspire, educate and enhance you.

- Take breaks! Daily, weekend and longer ones. If you feel the slightest sign of burn out, take a break!

- Don't think about all the reasons you can't and start thinking of all the ways you can!

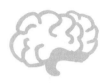

Chapter 6

CHANGE THE CONVERSATIONS WITH YOURSELF

I'm sure you've heard the saying, "watch your thoughts, they become your words and watch your words, they become your actions".

We talk to ourselves everyday. Why is that? Because you're the only one who really wants to listen to yourself all day. Lol. Okay kind of joking.

But seriously, we're talking to ourselves everyday, almost all day. Some things we say are positive, some of what we tell ourselves are just statements. If you recorded for a full month all of your self talk, you might be surprised how much of it negative self-talk trying to keep you still and silent.

Sometimes the voices in our heads are making sure we don't succeed. It's amazing how the one person we're supposed to trust, ourselves, is the one person keeping us from moving forward with our goals.

Autosuggestion is a way to repeat positive reinforcement to yourself to reprogram your sub-conscious. Say to yourself out loud, "I am loved. I am great. I have so much to offer to the world. I live in a world of peace, happiness and perfection." Was comfortable to say to yourself out loud? A little uncomfortable, right?

Now I want you to repeat this out loud to yourself: "This sucks! Things will never work out right!" Is that a little easier to say? Why does that come easily?

That just goes to show you that the "noises of the past" can become more comfortable to us. We become more accustomed to the negativity than the positive things in our head. This is why it's so important that we constantly auto suggest, and fill our sub-conscious brain with more positive thoughts. Through saying more positive things to ourselves, we counteract the noises.

It's never a perfect road to creating a better life and better "you". You see, before you can build yourself into the best version of you or before you can help others around you, you first have to address how you feel about "you" and overcome common roadblocks in your life.

Once you address this you then begin to realize that things will never be a perfect situation but you can still change history.

The problem exists when we want the situation to change but haven't changed our own course of direction. Your struggles of the past can become a distant memory if you begin to follow a different roadmap. Fear of the unknown and fear of change are what often keeps us from changing directions.

Sometimes the best thing you can do is something completely different than you're used to. What if you put yourself out there so much that you risk getting hurt, risk disappoint, risk what people say about you?

Be brave, be fierce and YOU dictate how the conversation goes. You're in control of your destiny.

In this chapter I'm going to give you a case study that highlights the notion that conversations with ourselves may be the cause of our situations. The following conversation is between myself and a client that I have worked with for some time. You will see that negative conversations ultimately kept her fat.

KAREN'S STORY

Karen is a working mother of two boys. She worked in Corporate America and raised one of her sons on her own until she got remarried. Karen battled with her weight most of her life all the way up until she turned

57. At 57, Karen met me and together we re-programmed her, mentally as well as physically. This changed her life. Today Karen enjoys being sixty pounds lighter, stronger and healthier. But as you'll see, it was a life long battle for her until she started applying all the concepts that you're learning in this book. Karen re-programmed her brain.

Karen said, "For me, I wasn't honest with myself. I knew I was overweight again, and I just would not come clean that I was overweight. I was in bigger clothes than I ever wore before. I wouldn't look in a mirror...ever." Karen didn't want to face her weight because she knew what she looked like, and didn't like the person staring back. Karen remembered a specific time when she got disgusted with herself. "I was in a pair of shorts with a tee shirt and I was in my dining room cleaning. I looked up, and we have a mirror in there, and I wondered who that person was in the mirror; because it wasn't me. And that was hard."

It's sometimes more painful to face a situation and do something about it, than rather just avoid it and not deal with it. It's easy to avoid, because you don't know what to do and you tried every diet. Karen had been up and down. In her 40's and 50's she kept putting on weight. She tried diets like Nutri-system again and again. She would do it for a couple weeks, and would just stop. Is this story familiar to you? You made some attempts, but they were not successful; they're short-lived. You didn't see the results right away and didn't lose those ten pounds in a month like they advertised, so you failed. You're easily discouraged.

You are told that you would lose ten pounds in a month and you didn't lose the ten pounds, and so you're in denial. Karen recalls," I knew I wasn't healthy. I can still see that image in the mirror. I just couldn't do it; I was just frozen in my life, and it was easier than to just buy the next size clothes. I had every size of clothing in my closet, so it was easier to just move up. You get it in your head: (this is going to be the way it is. Just deal with it.)"

You don't have to deal with it! You deserve better. You deserve to look your best and feel your best. Other conversations with yourself include thinking: "I'm too old, or it's too late and it's too hard. I haven't worked out in forever." So, it's easier not to do anything. You're getting a lot of different information from T.V. and from advertisements. All of those books and DVD's that promise you're going to lose ten pounds in ten months just sit on the bookshelf, right? Like I said before, you're receiving a lot of information but it still does not address the core issue which is reprogramming your brain to make the right decisions.

WHEN DID YOU FIRST START PUTTING ON WEIGHT?

Karen: "Oh. I was a fat kid, 200 pounds in eighth grade. I was the one they named animals after. Doctors back then, years and years and years ago, put me on diet pills, which were speed; so, I lost weight as a kid. But it was diet pills, there was no diet."

Greg: How did you get that heavy as a kid?

Karen: "I was big boned, I figured. I was the one that did the sneaking of the food. Nobody in my family was fat, but I was the one behind closed doors, eating the junk food when nobody was looking."

Greg: And that started as a child?

Karen: "Yup, since I was a young kid."

Greg: Were you involved in any programs or activities as a kid?

Karen: "No."

Greg: Did you go out in the yard and play?

Karen: "Well, we'd sometimes go out in the yard and play and I bowled on Saturday mornings. That was what I did. I grew up in the 50's and girls didn't play sports, so, we bowled, and ran around outside. I was not involved in any program for me to connect with other kids and form my own social circle."

Greg: Do you think as a kid, if you were more involved with positive social circles, it would have helped?

Karen: "I would guess, yes. I had my son in all of those programs and he always played sports; he always did stuff with kids after school. I came home from school and I ate, that's what I did. That was my thing, which today is still my big issue. I was the closet junk food junkie. It still haunts me. Getting on a schedule and eating meals is extremely important, and when I go off the reservation, I go back to the old way of sneaking the food."

Greg: So, the idle mind is the Devil's playground?

Karen: "Yes, that's it. For me, that's my thing. It's crucial to have somebody tell you what you can do and helping you; and nobody was there. I didn't know what to do. And then when I had to do something about it finally, I was forced to look. That was the thing that made me go to the gym."

Greg: That's when you looked to the right help.

Karen: "That was because I had to. You can be fat and you don't know. Nobody is telling you that you have to do something for your health; people will tell you very differently. You just buy another size clothes so you don't participate in things."

Greg: But the danger hasn't happened yet.

Karen: "No, the danger hasn't happened. So unless you have diabetes, or start getting high blood pressure, and then maybe that's when you go look for the help."

IT'S TOO LATE

Karen: "I honestly thought it was too late. I never thought I could do it. I never thought I could lose weight and be healthy."

Greg: So, the only thing that pushed you to the edge to move past that belief was that you ran into the health issues and the doctor told you that you had to do something? Essentially the doctor scared the crap out of you?

Karen: "Yes, the Doctor told me that I needed to change my life, and it still took me three months until I went to the gym from the moment he told me. I was still frozen in what to do. And I then had it in my mind that I had to lose weight and get healthy. I didn't believe that being strong was in the cards... until you told me we would get healthy first, and then we would get strong and lose weight. I still remember those words."

Greg: Now, sometimes when you're home, do you get that urge to go back to your old ways?

Karen: "Old ways, old habits."

Greg: What are some feelings that cause you to want to go back?

Karen: "Stress and comfort. Because that was the comfort. I mean, I know why I did what I did. I came home to an empty house, so I could justify it, but that was how I comforted myself. My mother was working and no other mothers worked, so I came home and I ate. So, when I have those feelings of loneliness or boredom, I look for food to comfort me."

Greg: Subconsciously.

Karen: "Oh, yeah."

Greg: It becomes automatic, without even thinking.

Karen: "Absolutely. It's an old habit that is familiar."

Greg: That's where the subconscious thinking comes in.

Karen: "Right. And it's a struggle to not do that and know that you can't do that. You can't go for the bag of potato chips. At some point I had to break the cycle."

Greg: That's your willpower. Your conscious mind is saying no, but your subconscious power is taking over. The automatic decision of grabbing for the potato chips can be reprogrammed. So, when you don't do that when you want to, you've begun to change a pattern. You've replaced that comfort with something else.

Karen: "Right. So, sometimes I'll go for a run. Sometimes I say, 'I have to come to the gym, because I don't want the old things to come back.' Sometimes I'll just make a cup of tea and go for a walk outside. But you have to do something to replace the negative behavior, and I know that now. So, it could even be cleaning or doing something around the house; but that feeling of 'I need this,' means I just have to do something else."

Greg: So in this Brain Detox Diet book, I name five noises in our head that we have to get rid of: Negativity, fear, distrust, anger and worry. And then, I came up with the six key motivators to replace those things: Reading, breathing, sleeping, moving, escaping and believing. So, you replaced some of the noises with moving.

Karen: "Yup, moving is important."

Greg: So now, instead of sitting home and eating a bag of potato chips...you get up and you go for a run.

Karen: "Yes!"

Greg: You've replaced it with one of the key motivators, moving. What about the other key motivators? Are you getting better with the sleeping?

Karen: "I've honestly made sleep a priority."

Greg: Breathing has always been a focus for you?

Karen: "Yes"

Greg: Because you've always had trouble breathing, you're aware of it; you're focusing on that.

Karen: "You have to replace the 'noises' you speak about: you have to do all six key motivators."

Greg: "It sounds like believing was a struggle for you. You felt held back until you turned 57 and received scary health news."

Karen: "Yup."

Greg: "Once you started training, I remember the story of reaching your first goal, which was to be able to wrap the towel around you after the shower."

Karen: "Wrap the towel, yes."

Greg: Tell us about that moment.

Karen: "In the gym, every woman would be in the locker room with a towel around them and I couldn't get it around me. I remember thinking 'There must be two size towels and I was using the small towel.' It was a couple weeks in when I realized it's the same towel, it just doesn't fit me. And so my goal was to wrap the towel around myself. I remember telling you that was my goal and I remember when it happened and I did it. I came out one day and said 'Guess what, I met my goal', and you looked at me with pride and that was an important moment. That, and then buying a pair of jeans that didn't have an elastic waist. That was moment number two."

Greg: Then you really believed.

Karen: "When I bought jeans without an elastic waist, I felt like I was on my way. But then there's more, it's not just the weight; it's all the other things you push your body to do. It's the mental part, doing things that people told you your whole life you couldn't do and then believing that you can do it and then looking at people and saying 'I can do it'!"

Greg: What about escaping? Is the gym an escape for you?

Karen: "Yeah. It's the one stable aspect of my life."

Greg: Especially Saturday mornings?

Karen: "Saturday mornings are important. It sets the tone for the week."

Greg: That's one of your key motivators.

Karen: "When I don't get to the gym, it's hard for me to keep my balance."

Greg: And it's more than that workout, right? It's also being around other people that are trying to do the same thing that you're trying to do; and the hellos and positive energy.

Karen: "When you do these kind of things, your friends don't change, but they don't necessarily understand unless they do it. So, coming to a gym that has people who all have the same focus is key. You have people who are doing it and rooting you on. There's no judgment, but every time you do something more, people recognize it. Your friends don't, your family doesn't, and you have to be able to deal with that. However, by coming to a gym, where everybody is in it together, it makes a big difference. And everybody knows how hard it is, that's why it's great to be there."

Greg: So there were people in your life that didn't get it at first. When you were eating differently and going to the gym more, you were probably getting some opposition from people, right?

Karen: "I did."

Greg: What did you do to set boundaries?

Karen: "Well, when I started really doing this, my best friend said 'Does this mean we're not going to be able to go out and party?' I had to explain that it's not about partying; it's about knowing how to live my life. You accept that people may not understand what you're doing. Your family and friends may be supportive, but they don't really get it the way people at the gym do. There's a difference between supporting and understanding."

Greg: Keeping your energy sacred.

I DON'T HAVE TIME

Let me tell you about Lisa. Lisa is a mom of 2 kids and works a 9-5 job. She's also married to Bill who commutes into the city for work so he is out of the house by 7am and doesn't get home until around 7pm.

I am sure Lisa is a lot like you. You're up early and you have to wake up the kids and then get ready for school, but they just don't want to move! Why is it on the weekends it seems like they're up so early yet when you have to get them going all they want do is sleep!

You're rushing to get them ready, pack lunches and maybe make them a quick bowl of cereal. Meanwhile you're trying to get yourself ready for your day. Even when you have some time for yourself, you're still thinking of a million things you have to do.

Plus, after work you have doctor appointments, kids practice and maybe an extra conference call. You say: "screw the gym, I need a drink." And speaking of the gym...when you do actually make it for a workout, there's not much time so you say: "let me skip the warm up" and "oh, I've got to skip this part of my workout because I have somewhere to be." Bottom line, your workout suffers!

Does this sound familiar so far?

But lately, pounds have been adding up and you're feeling unmotivated and sluggish. And you may even be struggling in the intimacy department. Besides...who has time for that, you're so busy!

The reason you tell yourself that you have no time is...

You put everything before YOU!

You put your jobs, your kids, your spouse (sometimes), your friends, your favorite TV show. Now I know these are all very important to you, but YOU are very important. Without taking care of YOU and putting yourself first, everything else will eventually suffer because you will not be at your best, both physically and mentally.

Don't worry, you're not being selfish. Actually, your kids, your spouse, your friends and the world are counting on you to be your best. If you don't make the time to just focus on you and your health, then you will drop the ball on everything you work so hard to accomplish.

BE VERY CAREFUL OF MIND TRAPS

Be careful of the traps your mind sets. It's very easy to fall into the trap your mind sets when you're trying to achieve something significant. This can be anything from losing a lot of weight, starting or growing a business or completing any goal for that matter.

Here's the scenario...you have a vision of this big goal you want to accomplish. You get started with moving towards this goal and you're very excited in the beginning. Shortly after beginning, the obstacles start coming at you and it gets harder and harder to stay excited and focused. After a short time working on this big goal you're still not seeing any results and it's starting to look like it's going to take forever. Discouragement sets in big time! It almost feels not worth the trouble and work anymore. "Why am I even attempting this? I'm not going to be able to do this. Forget it, it's impossible."

This is a mind trap.

I want to help you not to fall for these traps and teach you how. Lately I took on a new hobby that I do on quiet week nights. My new hobby as of late is putting together puzzles. These are not just any puzzles though, they are the hard ones: 1000pc puzzles. If you ever tried to put together a 1000pc puzzle you'll see how hard they are. These puzzles take a lot of patience. Here's where the lesson came to me that made a lot of sense. Think of your big goal like finishing the 1000pc puzzle. At first you're excited to get started to put this puzzle together, but almost immediately after starting you realize that you have 1000 things to put together and the progress is very slow, especially in the beginning. You can easily get caught up in the trap of getting frustrated because after some time of putting pieces together, you still can't see the finished product.

When you have a big goal or vision don't get caught up in the fact that you're not close enough to the finished product. Stay focused on putting a few pieces together at a time. The finished product will come, but you have to shrink it down and knock out one part or section at a time. Take your time and be patient. Next thing you know, you will gain momentum and those scattered 1000 pieces will start to take shape and show results. You have your vision of the final product. Now just focus on one piece of the puzzle at a time and remember to enjoy the process of piecing it together.

Whatever your personal battle or fight is, there is something you can do right now to stand proud. That's to get up and keep fighting. You can't lose the fight if you keep getting up! One day a very overweight and timid girl stepped into my gym with her parents. Her name was Carrie. Carrie had been through the ringer and looked defeated. She was severely picked on and bullied most of her life and this fight eventually kept her down. Until one day, She got up!

And fought back.

Carrie had a huge hurdle in front of her: lose all the weight and get in shape. Everyday Carrie showed up and kept fighting. Carrie will tell you, there were more days she can count that she was exhausted and knocked down. But Carrie kept getting up and kept fighting! So much so, that we nicknamed her "The Terminator." You have to be the terminator in life. It doesn't matter how many blows you've taken, get up and keep fighting!

Today Carrie is 100lbs. lighter, in great shape and is one of my valued employees now. During her journey Carrie got certified as a personal trainer and now helps other people achieve their best.

I know the blows hurt. Shake it off, get up and keep fighting. The bell hasn't rung yet!

GREG'S PIA'S (Put Into Action)

- Whichever area in your life you need help in, find a qualified and recommended coach to help you and design a plan to improve.

- Don't let roadblocks and setbacks discourage you. Anything worth fighting for takes time, work and faith.

- Stay focus on the Brain Detox properties and your mindset will improve.

- If you're having a bad day, week, month or year; don't let that stop you from achieving your dreams. The harder and darker the storm, the brighter the sun shines once it's over... and it's right around the corner.

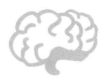

Chapter 7

THE STRESS FREE DIET

Now that you started your brain detox, you should be able to use your inner strength and focus to stick with any healthy diet. I'm going to introduce you to a way to eat and look at food differently. This will enable you to stay lean all year round stress free. Food should be viewed as a way to nourish your body and give it the proper nutrients to perform. Most people can't maintain their diet because it becomes too stressful and this causes them to backslide. Dieting should not be stressful, it should be a way of life. The diet you choose to follow should fit your lifestyle.

I've been coaching clients for a long time and have come across many different ways to lose weight and drop body fat. Every time I hear the question, "what diet works the best?" I can't help but say to myself... The one that you can stick to.

There are a hundred different diets and theories out there as to which is the best for having a lean body. And they're ALL good! They ALL can work at getting you leaner. So for you, it has to be the best one for YOU. That one YOU can stick to. THE STRESS FREE DIET.

So what does this mean? That you can do the "hamburger and french fries diet" and still lose weight? NO! It means if eating 5-6 small meals a day is going to stress you out to the point of giving up, than that's not for you. Getting the same nutrients in 4 meals might be more your speed.

If trying to never eat grains again is going to cause you to binge than that's not for you. Eating grains at the right time (like meals after intense workouts so your body doesn't store it all as fat,) may be what helps you succeed.

It's all about giving your body what it needs at the right times in the right amounts and nothing more. You have to choose a diet that makes sense for you and that you will be able to maintain over a period of time. Dieting to lose weight or lean out is about consistency, not trying something out for two weeks.

It's about lifestyle and good habits, NOT WILLPOWER. Wills are easily broken. It's important to remember...if something isn't working for you, it's time to change it.

THE BIG FOUR HORMONES AND NEUROTRANSMITTERS

This section is going to bring all the previous chapters together because everything you learned in those chapters is designed to improve the big four hormones and neurotransmitters. Let's first talk about what the big four hormones and neurotransmitters are and what they do. Both control many functions and feelings in your body that have to do with weight control. Neurotransmitters are the "feel good" chemicals that send signals to your brain and have a major impact on mood, feelings and behaviors. Your hormones are chemicals transported by the bloodstream to other parts of the body, with the intent of influencing a variety of physiological and behavioral activities. These activities include: processes of digestion, metabolism, growth, reproduction, mood and weight control. Both can be improved by following the brain detox diet principles.

NEUROTRANSMITTERS

An imbalance or low levels of these neurotransmitters cause many food addictions and emotional eating. Sugar and carbohydrates will give you an initial spike in dopamine and serotonin, which is why some people turn to those types of feel good foods. The good feeling is short lived and those feel good chemicals in your brain dip fast. Another adverse side effect is that the more you do this, the weaker the reaction of the chemical becomes, so you begin to eat more junk food to find that good feeling again. This is how addictions are formed. Let's take a look at the big four neurotransmitters.

1. Dopamine

One of the neurotransmitters playing a major role in addiction is **dopamine**. Many of the concepts that apply to dopamine apply to other neurotransmitters as well. As a chemical messenger, dopamine is similar to adrenaline. Dopamine affects brain processes that control movement, emotional response, and ability to experience pleasure and pain. It also acts as our reward sensation chemical, so you can see how certain food addictions could develop because of low levels of dopamine.

How do you naturally increase dopamine without binge eating? Dopamine uses the amino acid Tyrosine to be produced. Eating foods high in this amino acid, like chicken, fish, turkey, avocados, bananas and some soy products, will increase dopamine. Also, go back to your **6 key motivators,** especially moving and sleeping. Just a side note- sex would be in the moving category and has been known to be great for dopamine levels! Lastly, focusing on healthy reward systems when reaching new goals will do the trick. Since dopamine is a reward chemical you will want to mimic that. Like sticking to a very healthy and clean diet all week and treating yourself on a Saturday night to some dessert and a glass of wine.

2. Serotonin

Serotonin is better known as the "feel good" chemical. This neurotransmitter tends to be low when we suffer from depression. This is why so many doctors are prescribing antidepressants that serve to increase your serotonin levels. Turning to food can temporarily give you a boost, but that is short lived. So, besides medication, some natural ways to turn up the serotonin and get us out of the blues is through diet, exercise, frequent physical contact and using some of the other key motivators like sleeping, breathing and moving.

Eating a diet that is high in DHA, or better known as omega-3 fatty acids, is known to have an effect on our production of serotonin. This includes: fish, almonds, avocados and flaxseed. These are all staples of the stress free diet.

Next is exercise and moving. Keeping your body in motion with some high intensity exercise helps to balance the scale and boost the "feel good" chemicals. Human contact on a regular basis is also important. It is said that babies need constant human contact in order to develop normally. Well that doesn't stop as an adult! It is in our nature to need to feel physical contact regularly, as it has an effect on our hormonal and brain chemical makeup. This can come from frequent hugs, pats on the shoulders, sex, or even frequent massages. Finally let's add a dose of the two Key Motivators, sleeping and breathing, for the final boost. By following all the advice laid out for you in this book, you should start to find relief if you do suffer from depression.

3. Gaba

While there is more scientific information on the neurotransmitter **gaba**, I'm going to keep this one short and sweet since it's not as popularly known to impact weight loss. It does; however, have a role in muscle tone. Its first use during childhood is for development of the brain, but as we age, inhibited levels of Gaba have an effect on muscle tone and motor neuron control. Gaba cannot be supplemented but is synthesized from both the amino acid Glutamine and vitamin B6, both which can be supplemented. Normal levels of Gaba are known to have a calming effect on the central nervous system.

4. Endorphins

This is the fun neurotransmitter! Produced in the pituitary gland of the brain, **endorphins** control excitement and acts as a painkiller in the body. This is another "feel good" chemical. Sometimes working together with the chemical, adrenaline, you mostly get peaks of endorphins in your blood level during rigorous exercise or sometimes during trauma to block pain. (Obviously we want to trigger this more during exercise.) Not only exercise can trigger endorphins flowing through the body, but also other mood enhancing outside factors can give us this rush. One of these outside factors can be particular foods. Be mindful of this. For someone who is not overly active, food can be your endorphin trigger that will result in eating issues. Find your endorphin rush from exercise, daily activities and other healthy factors in life that just excite you and make you feel good.

SUGAR ADDICTION

Sugar happens to be one of the main culprits that give you an initial rush of these four neurotransmitters I just detailed for you. As previously mentioned, it becomes addicting when sugar gives you a quick release of feel good chemicals in the body. However, I will reiterate: this is short lived. It then becomes a vicious cycle of eating more and more sugar based foods to get feel good chemicals back in. Am I scaring you yet? Good!

Question: Would you survive longer on a diet of just water OR on a diet of water and refined sugar? Answer: You would survive longer on just water. Five sailors who were ship wrecked in 1793 helped to prove this answer. The ship was filled with sugar, thus giving the marooned five a diet of sugar and water. When they were finally picked up nine days later, they were in a wasted condition due to starvation.

The story of the five sailors intrigued French physiologist Francois Magendie to conduct a series of experiments in which he fed dogs a diet of sugar. All of the dogs died. Magendie proved that as a steady diet, refined sugar is worse than having nothing. How can sugar be worse than nothing? Plainly put, refined sugar is an anti-nutrient. It starts out as sugar cane, and then goes through an extensive refining process that destroys all of the enzymes, fiber, vitamins and minerals. What you're left with are empty calories. The problem is that your body needs the enzymes, fiber, vitamins and minerals that were taken out in the refining process in order to metabolize sugar and use it as energy. So it takes those nutrients from your own body. So while you are enjoying that chocolate bar, sugar is draining vital nutrients from your body. Sugar creates false hunger (as a result of the insulin rush and then ensuing plummet in your blood sugar levels), which makes you overeat. This means a constant struggle with your weight in which you never seem to achieve your ideal size. Sugar promotes aging due to the advanced glycation end products, or AGEs, that occur when insulin levels are consistently elevated as a result of eating too much sugar. Sugar has even been dubbed "the negative fountain of youth."

Sugar weakens your bones, making you vulnerable for osteoporosis. It also weakens your teeth, making you vulnerable for cavities (due to the calcium being pulled from your bones and teeth in order for your body to process sugar).

Sugar in excess is stored as fat. After your liver has no more room to store sugar, it is converted to fat and deposited in your belly, thighs, hips and the backs of your arms. Sugar can impair brain functioning as a result of depleted B-vitamin production.

If you're still not convinced of the danger of sugar here are more ailments linked to its overconsumption: varicose veins, constipation, hormonal imbalances, ADD and ADHD, increased emotional instability, depressed immune system, increased risk of cancer and degenerative diseases.

The average modern person consumes approximately 46 teaspoons of sugar every day. That comes out to roughly 175 pounds of sugar each year. It's no wonder that the sugar industry is big business!

Go through the foods in your home and you'll see that sugar has been added to everything from ketchup and spaghetti sauce to crackers, oatmeal, peanut butter and even 'healthy' items like weight loss bars. While all other foods offer you caloric energy PLUS some nutritional benefit, sugar does not. Sugar is simply caloric energy with a sweet habit forming taste, and a hoard of health risks.

THE MANY NAMES OF SUGAR

While you're checking out nutrition labels for sugar content be on the lookout for the following names that all describe refined sugar: Sucrose, High fructose corn, syrup, Fructose, Lactose, Organic sugar, Maltose, Dextrose and Glucose.

HORMONES

Once we have an understanding of the chemicals in the brain that control some of our eating habits it's crucial that we also have a good understanding of the four big hormones, which really have a huge impact on our body types, weight control and our moods.

Hormones are defined as biochemicals produced in particular parts of organisms by specific cells, glands, and/or tissues and then transported by the bloodstream to other parts of the body. Hormones have the intent of influencing a variety of physiological and behavioral activities. These include the processes of digestion, metabolism, growth, reproduction, and mood control. Your big four hormones really tell the story of your body: which you may be deficient in, which hormone might be over produced and which hormone needs to be controlled better. Sometimes we need to take a look at a person's hormonal situation before even addressing their diet. Without proper balance of these hormones, your body will not respond properly no matter what you eat.

If you haven't lately, it would probably be a good idea to get some blood work done and have a doctor take a look at your levels of the big four. Here is what to look for: DHEA, Testosterone, Estradiol- (Main female sex hormone and byproduct of testosterone metabolism,) Cortisol, IGF-1 (Growth hormone surrogate) and TSH (thyroid activity.)

1. Testosterone

When you think about testosterone, the first thing you probably think of is a hormone making men big, muscular and hairy. You'll be surprised that this hormone is not only important for men but for women as well. Women have a much lower level of testosterone, but we all need it.

Testosterone is an anabolic and sex hormone, which is responsible for sexual desire and function, reproduction, muscular hypertrophy, strong bones, and hair growth. This hormone is especially important in terms of keeping both men <u>and</u> women lean. In fact, most people are very low in the hormone due to current environmental factors, poor diets and chronic stress. Cortisol is a popular stress hormone that is becoming very common, as it is wreaking havoc on our health and testosterone levels. High levels of cortisol are on the rise due to chronic stress. Many people are suffering from increased stress and cortisol works against testosterone causing you to hold onto fat much easier. It's important that we address this issue in both men _and_ women. Women, like men, are showing dangerous signs of high cortisol levels and decreased testosterone. The good news is we can do something about it. There are changes we can make and actions we can take to lower cortisol and naturally raise testosterone to normal levels for both men and women. We can do this by changing our lifestyles.

Here are my recommendations:

- Increase lifting weights that actually push you to 10-15 rep max. This should not be easy!
- Be cautious of only doing long endurance cardio. This has been showed, at times, to over stress the body and raise cortisol levels. Instead break it up with high intensity interval cardio mixed with rest periods. (Yes, actually rest and bring your heart rate down before your next interval!)
- Eat natural, unsaturated fats from eggs, fish, nuts and oils.
- Increase your protein intake and supplement with whey protein powder and BCAA (Branched Chain Amino Acids) capsules.
- Supplement with plenty of antioxidants (We will cover that shortly in this book)
- Stay moving.

- Sleep more.
- Have plenty of sex.
- Do your breathing exercises.

2. Estrogen

Estrogen is better known as the female hormone. Estrogen is also found in males as well. Testosterone aromatizes or gets synthesized into estrogen, which can be one of the causes for men getting what's commonly known as "man boobs." Usually when a man holds onto fat at the pec/chest region, it's a sign that his testosterone might be low.

Mostly everyone knows that estrogen is the hormone responsible for making a woman a "woman", as far as their traits and reproductive system are concerned. However, can too much estrogen make you more of a woman or fatter? According to an article in *Shape* magazine, it's often common for women in their 30's and 40's to have elevated estrogen levels, sometimes 3 to 4 times higher than normal. Numerous things can cause this, but diet and toxicity seem to play a major role. One sign that a woman suffers from elevated estrogen is when they tend to hold on to more fat around the hip, butt and legs. So if you're a woman, it may be a good idea to make sure your hormones land in a normal zone. One way to possibly balance out your hormone levels is to do all the things I detailed for you in the testosterone section. Don't worry, I promise you won't start growing a beard!

- Increase lifting weights that actually push you to 10-15 rep max. This should not be easy!
- Be cautious of with doing long endurance cardio. Instead break it up with high intensity interval cardio mixed with rest periods. Yes actually rest and bring your heart rate down before your next interval.
- Eat natural unsaturated fats from eggs, fish, nuts and oils.
- Increase your protein intake and supplement with whey protein powder and BCAA capsules.
- Supplement with plenty of antioxidants (We will cover that shortly in this book)
- Stay moving.
- Sleep more.
- Have plenty of sex.
- Do your breathing exercises.

3. Insulin

Insulin is a necessary hormone in the body, which regulates blood sugar. It is also known as our fat storing hormone. When our blood stream is filled with sugar from carbohydrates, insulin is released to lower the volume of sugar in the blood and allow the sugar to be used or stored. The problem arises when too much insulin response happens in the body due to consumption of excess amounts of sugar at one time causing storage in our fat cells. This needs to be regulated better. Another name for this is *insulin sensitivity*. Someone who stores fat easily tends to be more insulin sensitive because any time they eat food that contains carbohydrates or sugar, they release insulin right away. We want to become more efficient at using this sugar (glucose) as energy or to store it in our muscle and liver, not as body fat.

I want you to picture your body as one big fuel tank. You have storage containers in your muscles and a storage container in your liver. Now picture your arteries as the tubes that connect all of your storage containers. Now, the sugar, carbohydrates and even fats and proteins are the gas/fuel. (But for this scenario we'll focus more on the carbohydrates and sugars.) Now, picture in your head pouring the gas/fuel into your body, which goes into your storage tanks. First, it starts to fill up your liver and that fills up quickly since there's not much to hold there. Next, it starts filling up the storage tanks that make your muscles, and unless you have large muscle tanks, they begin to fill up quickly. Next thing you know, all tanks are full at capacity, so you have gas/fuel spilling over and filling up your artery tubes. This is where insulin comes in. Your body responds by releasing insulin into the body to move that overflow of sugar/gas/fuel into a new storage unit that can keep building and building. Yes you guessed it; this is your body fat!

This is why it's beneficial to eat a diet with a lower carbohydrate intake, or when we do eat foods that contain carbohydrates, eat the ones that have a lower glycemic index. This means they have a slower release of sugar into the bloodstream, or your storage tank tubes. You ultimately want it to look more like a hospital IV rather than pumping gas at the gas station. Make sense? Also, the better shape you are in and the better diet you have (less refined carbs and higher protein) will reduce your insulin sensitivity. Your body will not release insulin as quickly, which will result in less fat storage.

4. Growth Hormone

This is the "fountain of youth" hormone. Growth hormone is called this because it plays a large role in keeping us young by keeping us strong, keeping our metabolisms fast, keeping our skin tight, and keeping our hair and nails growing. As we age, natural growth hormone that is released starts to diminish. Lowered growth hormone release also happens with people that suffer from an inactive thyroid or hypothyroidism because the thyroid is the gland that is involved with growth hormone release.

Growth hormone is usually released optimally during REM sleep and small amounts during rigorous exercise like lifting heavier weights.

WHERE DO YOU HOLD YOUR WEIGHT? WHICH HORMONE IS LINKED TO THIS AND WHAT CAN WE DO ABOUT IT?

- Hips, butt and legs = Elevated estrogen = Toxicity
  o Eat organic.
  o Take out processed foods and preservatives/chemicals.
  o Supplementation.
  o Stay away from soy products.
  o Increase sleep.

- o Incorporate high intensity exercise and full body movements.
- Love handles and stomach = High refined carb diet
  - o No refined carbs/breads.
  - o Eat less grains.
  - o Eat vegetables.
  - o Lower alcohol intake.
  - o Increase proteins and fats.

- Extended stomach only = High cortisol = Stress
  - o Increase sleep.
  - o Reduce sugar and alcohol intake.
  - o Read.
  - o Breathing/meditation techniques.
  - o Escaping.
  - o Organization and Preparation.

- Back of arms and chest = Low testosterone
  - o Increase protein and unsaturated fat intake.
  - o Supplementation.
  - o High intensity exercise.
  - o Increase sleep.

DETOX AND BALANCE THE BODY

Before I talk about the macronutrients of the stress free diet, which contains proteins, fats and carbohydrates, I want to discuss micronutrients are that are important to keep our bodies in balance and free from toxicity. These micronutrients are vitamins, minerals and antioxidants. Every function of the body down to a cellular level starts with vitamins, minerals and antioxidants. Why is this important? Most people lack the right amount or balance of these nutrients. This lack or imbalance often becomes the root cause of many health and weight loss issues. Unfortunately, because of the modernized world, our bodies are bombarded with toxins daily and depleted from nutrients in the food we eat. So it's our responsibility to make sure we are taking proper steps in order to get the right amounts of nutrients in our bodies. This will help us function properly and fight off certain diseases. Besides eating a very clean diet of whole foods cooked correctly, the other step to take is through supplementation. In this section I will explain the function of all three micronutrients and then give you my list of the top micronutrients to be aware of.

Antioxidants protect each and every individual cell from a toxic environment. They especially protect us from free radicals. Free radicals are highly unstable molecules that seek out other molecules in your body and steal the electron they are missing from that molecule. This process results in the injury and eventual death of the cell. Now multiply this process times a billion and you see the danger it poses to your body. Your body can only be as healthy as the sum of its cells. If many of your body's cells are unhealthy and dying from free radical attacks then your overall health and vitality will be drastically lowered. The good news is that free radicals are not a problem if your body is full of antioxidants. The antioxidant neutralizes the free radical. This shows the great importance of constantly replenishing your body's supply of antioxidants.

Vitamins are essential for growth, vitality and health, and are helpful in digestion, elimination, and resistance to disease. Depletions or deficiencies can lead to a variety of both specific nutritional disorders and general health problems, depending on which vitamin is lacking in the diet. Minerals are just as important as vitamins and sometimes harder to get since there are only trace amounts found in the foods we eat. We are all made up of minerals, which are elements that come from the earth. Minerals are essential to our physical and mental health. Let's take a look at some of the more important micronutrients that I recommend you supplement with in order to create a stress free and more balanced environment for your body to work properly.

DETOX THE BODY WITH THESE POWERFUL ANTIOXIDANTS, VITAMINS, MINERALS AND SUPPLEMENTS:

1. Vitamin C

This is a water-soluble antioxidant, which is not produced by the body and must be obtained through food and supplementation. Vitamin C is a potent, free radical quencher and it is essential for a strong immune system. Studies show that people who take vitamin c supplements live longer, healthier lives than those who don't. Vitamin C recycles vitamin E, giving your immune system an added boost. Vitamin C also suppresses viruses in the body and strengthens connective tissue (particularly collagen, which keeps the skin tight and wrinkle free). For men especially, vitamin C is also involved with the health and strength of the arterial walls, having a major impact on cholesterol levels.

2. Vitamin E

This is the body's primary fat-soluble antioxidant. It, too, must be obtained from food or supplements. As an anti-aging antioxidant, vitamin E protects your skin against damage from UV radiation and ozone. Studies have also shown that vitamin E prevents heart disease, stroke and reduces the risk of certain cancers. The two forms of vitamin E are tocopherols and tocotrienols.

3. Lipoic Acid

This is known as the universal antioxidant. It can recycle all other antioxidants and raise levels of glutathione which is a powerful antioxidant, that when taken orally, is not well absolved by the body. Lipoic acid is critical for energy production because it helps break down sugar to be used by the cells and also protects the mitochondria (the "powerhouse" of the cell).

4. Flaxseed oil or fish oil (Omega 3)

Omega 3's (Fish Oil and High-lignan Flaxseed Oil) and Omega 6's (GLA or Evening Primrose Oil) are the unsaturated fats, which are needed in your body for many functions. These functions include:

- Mood Stabilization

Essential fats are used for brain function and production of certain mood stabilizing chemicals and hormones.

- Making the Heart Healthier

Omega 3 acts as a natural blood thinner. The heart is inarguably one of the most important parts of our body and having an unhealthy heart means having to suffer a rather limited lifespan. Naturally, it's in our best interest to keep our hearts happy and healthy and one way of doing that is eating food that contains fish oil. For instance, in Athens, Greece, a study was done to show the relationship between high fish diet and inflammation of blood vessels. The results revealed that the group who ate more fish than the other group had a lower level of C-reactive protein and interleukin-6, factors that are commonly used to measure likelihood of blood vessel inflammation. These benefits remained even when the various risks associated with high fish diet were taken into account.

- Fish to Become Thin

In Perth, Australia, a study had revealed that fish consumption could be used against hypertension and obesity.

Researchers of the "UWA" University of Western Australia have discovered that a weight-loss diet, which includes a regular amount of fish consumption, can be quite effective in reducing blood pressure and improving glucose tolerance.

- Fish Oil to Combat Asthma

People suffering from respiratory problems like asthma tend to be perceived as unfit and unhealthy. They should now be pleased to learn that certain studies have revealed the benefits of fish oil for asthma-burdened individuals. Statistics show that approximately 20 to 25% of children today suffer one form of asthma or another at a certain point in their lives. Certain evidence reveals a regular diet of food with high linoleic acid content as the reason behind this. Researchers of "UW" conducted a study by subjecting a number of children to a high-fish diet while others continued with their regular diet. Results revealed that the participants who ate more fish were less prone to asthma attacks and were able to breath more easily.

Essential fatty acids must always be part of our daily diet. Without them, we take one step closer to our deaths. Essential fatty acids are divided into two families: omega-6 EFAs and omega-3 EFAS. Although there are only very slight differences to distinguish the two groups of essential fatty acids from each other, studies have revealed that too much intake of omega-6 EFAs can lead to inflammation, blood clotting and tumor growth. The good news, however, is that the opposite is true for omega-3 EFAs. Omega-6 EFAs can be found in vegetable oils while omega-3 EFAs can be found in fish oils among other foods. Omega-6 vs. Omega-3 physicians and scientists are of the same opinion that the cause behind increasing cases of heart disease, high blood pressure, obesity, diabetes, premature aging and certain kinds of cancer is none other than an imbalanced intake of omega-3 and omega-6 EFAs.

As explored earlier, omega-6 EFAs can be found in vegetable oils. This includes but is not limited to corn oil and soy oil, both of which contains high amounts of linoleic acid. Omega-3 EFAs on the other hand can be found also in marine plankton and walnut and flaxseed oils. It should be significant to take note that fatty fish and fish oils contain eicosapentaenoic acid (EPA) and docosahexaenoic acid (DHA), fatty acids that have been observed to provide many benefits to the human body.

In the early 1970's, a study on Greenland Eskimos have revealed that one of the major reasons why they rarely suffer from heart diseases is because of their high-fat diet (mainly composed of fish). The eggs of salmon were dried and stored as an important item of nutrition for both children and adults. They were also used to increase the fertility in women. From a chemical standpoint, the oil from fish is one of the most nutritious foods anywhere. It was no wonder the primitive Eskimo were able to provide their bodies with all the nutrients they needed to survive under such extreme conditions. However, soon the westernized, modern diet would come and rapidly decrease this population causing more disease due to lack of nutrients and medical care. (Weston A. Price – Nutrition and physical degeneration)

The average modern diet is almost completely lacking in omega oils. For example, the majority of people in America are over 80% deficient in these essential oils. That is cause for serious concern. To make matters worse, the average diet provides much in the way of unhealthy, disease causing fats. Combine the deficient levels of Omega 3s with the over abundance of bad fats and you have a recipe for disease and rapid aging. The two essential fatty acids, EPA and DHA, are also helpful in preventing atherosclerosis, heart attacks, depression and various forms of cancer. Fish oil supplemented food has also proven to be useful in treating illnesses like rheumatoid arthritis, diabetes, Raynaud's disease and ulcerative colitis.

5. Multi green powders

Multi-vitamins or other supplements ensure that you are getting "good" nutritional insurance; however they tend to turn your urine a fluorescent color. Ever wonder why? The answer is your body is NOT absorbing the vitamins properly. Worse, some recent studies have indicated that synthetic vitamins may be detrimental to our health. Much of the synthetic multi's they sell in the stores pass right through you and don't contain everything you need on a daily basis, especially since the food we eat now is lacking in nutrients (from cooking it or growth in poor soil.) These new multi green powders are the way to go. Most of the nutrient dense powder comes from real organic sources of fruits and vegetables, so naturally your body can process this much better. Also, companies are now able to pack so many more important nutrients that we need into these powders without us having to go purchase another pill bottle for each one. I personally can feel the difference when I take my "green drink" compared to when I do not. As a matter of fact, I recently had a supplement and vitamin intervention with my brother. He was never much of a vitamin and supplement taker, but was complaining of a few health issues like sciatic nerve pain, low energy, mood swings and heartburn. After buying his first order of green powder and getting him to commit to taking it for at least thirty days, my brother called me to say how completely different he felt since drinking the powder consistently. Today he's hooked. There are a few good products out there so do your research and make sure they are organic or GMO free. My recommendation, (and I'm not affiliated with them but just use it myself) is a company called Athletic Greens. They ship it to me every month with a new monthly batch. It contains almost everything I mention in this book.

6. Vitamin D3

Humans have the ability to synthesize Vitamin D from skin exposure to the sun. Ancestral humans evolved with continual exposure to sunlight. Unfortunately, 50% of today's Americans have been shown to be clinically deficient in this essential vitamin. Conservative estimates place our needed levels at 15,000 to 20,000 IU of Vitamin D per day. Studies have shown that best form of oral Vitamin D is Vitamin D3. The research on the benefits of

Vitamin D is overwhelming and it may be one of the most important supplements you can take to ward off a wide range of physical, emotional and neurological diseases. Some of the benefits include:

- Fight obesity and Type 2 Diabetes.
- Maintain healthy bone and prevent osteoporosis.
- Fight Alzheimer's and other neuro-degenerative diseases.
- Improve Blood Pressure.
- Defend against Autoimmune Diseases like Fibromyalgia and Psoriasis.
- Improve Moods, Alleviate Depression and Chronic Fatigue Syndrome.
- Reduce the Risk of Breast, Prostate and Colon Cancers.
- Boost muscle strength and boost fertility.

7. Green Tea

EGCG found in green tea may block the mutation of cells and reduce cell damage. It may also block the liver enzymes that convert pro-carcinogens into carcinogens (harmful cells)

Scientists have revealed that green tea is 10-100 times more potent than black tea and can block enzymes that cause cancer cells to grow. Tea increases the blood's antioxidant capacity. Green tea has been shown to reduce damage to blood vessels in smokers. Green tea's polyphenols can boost white blood cells, and might be an effective supplement to chemotherapy and radiation treatments that impact bone marrow and lower white blood cell count. A cup of green tea may provide 10-40mg of polyphenols and has antioxidant activity greater than a serving of broccoli, spinach, carrots or strawberries.

8. Vitamin B complex

This is also water-soluble and can be taken more frequently because the B vitamins are not stored in the liver. The B complex vitamin contains the right balance of all the b vitamins. This balance is important because all the B vitamins work synergistically together. When taking more than 100 mg of lipoic acid, more B vitamin biotin is needed because they can compete with each other. The B vitamins are needed for things ranging from energy production, regulation of cholesterol and prevention of birth defects.

9. Magnesium/zinc

Magnesium strengthens bones and teeth, it promotes healthy muscle contractions, and is important for the heart muscle and nervous system. It is essential for energy production in the body. Magnesium also acts as a natural muscle relaxer and calms nerve conduction when taken at night before bed.

Zinc is a component in over 200 enzymes in the body. Zinc is essential for growth, healing and control of hormones from organs such as the testes and ovaries. Zinc also aids in the ability to cope with stress effectively and support the immune system.

10. BCAA's (Branched Chains Amino Acids)

Among the most beneficial and effective supplements in any sports nutrition program are branched chain amino acids. These include the essential aminos leucine, iso-leucine, and valine. The essential branched chain amino acids (BCAA's) are of special importance for athletes because they are metabolized in the muscle, rather than in the liver. Here's how this works: After digestion, once protein is broken down into individual amino acids, these aminos can either be used to build new proteins or be burned as fuel to produce energy. Amino acids are the building blocks of protein. When you eat a protein rich food, it gets digested in the stomach and intestine into individual amino acids and short chains of amino acids that are small enough to be absorbed into the bloodstream. These amino acids have far reaching effects in the body from building tissues, to producing chemicals that enable our brains to function optimally.

INTERMITTENT FASTING AND CLEANSING

This type of dieting is gaining some popularity in the world of health and fitness. It typically consists of getting all your nutrients in with fewer meals. It allows for some cheat meals to create a non-plateau environment, and is followed by a day of fasting. You typically eat 3-4 meals between an 8-hour period. This allows you to eat a heartier serving of nutrients and less meals in the day, which can make eating less stressful. Also, one of the goals with this type of dieting is to decrease insulin sensitivity. As I mentioned in the section on hormones, the less insulin we release the better, because of it's fat storage properties.

Cleanses and detox drinks have become popular, which I favor to a point. I think there's a time and place for these and too much of anything is not a good thing. My opinion is that every now and then a good two-day cleanse is good for the body. It will detox your body and reset your digestive system while flooding the body with nutrients. The sample meal plan I lay out in this book includes a semi-fast and detox drink once a week after your cheat meal day.

WHY YOUR DIET SHOULD CONSIST OF HIGH PROTEIN AND VEGETABLE/ MODERATE FATS AND LOW CARBS

This should be the format for your diet. It really comes down to knowing when and what types of foods to eat. I just finished naming all our important vitamins, minerals and nutrients. The following diet will provide you with a nice balance of the above. Vegetables, which contain the most vitamins and minerals, are the staple of the stress free diet. You can't have enough vegetables full of nutrients, especially those dark green leafy ones. The second main component is protein-based food. This should be the second thing you eat on your plate. The main sources of protein should come from fish, chicken, eggs and some red meat. Protein is the building block of keeping your body strong and lean whether you are a woman or a man. Most proteins contain some amount of fat, but don't be afraid of fat from proteins. You want to use fats as a primary source of energy. Unsaturated fat or fat from animal protein packs more fuel per gram than carbohydrates do. Our bodies want to use fat for energy before carbohydrates, so when you eat a meal that contains proteins, fats and carbs, the carbohydrates are usually the last to be used as energy and thus stored in the body as fat. Complex carbs or grains are beneficial only after rigorous training, weight lifting and sprinting. So eat them only in meals after those types of work-outs to replenish glycogen stores (stored energy in the muscles). Remember the section on insulin and how our muscles are the storage tanks? Carbohydrates give us that full feeling and that's why it gets hard to reduce our intake, so timing when you eat them is important and will make more sense when it comes to an eating plan.

Vegetarians* If you're a vegetarian, it's important that you find other ways of getting adequate amounts of protein in your diet. I have had some vegetarian clients that will eat eggs and some that don't. In my opinion, eggs are the perfect food for weight control. They contain all essential amino acids making it the perfect protein, plus a good source of good omega 3 fats with the yolk.

SCHEDULING AND PREPARING YOUR MEALS

This is probably one of the most important parts of a sound diet. Without being prepared and having a meal schedule it will be very easy to fall off track and go back to old bad habits. I can't emphasize this part enough. Maintaining an eating schedule and being prepared with most of your meals is just as important as the food you eat. Take out your appointment book. Now schedule your meals around meetings, kids stuff, workouts and anything else in your day. Your eating plan should be as consistent as brushing your teeth. You should know each day about what time you eat each meal and snack so that it's consistent and you don't forget to eat. Some days will not be perfect, but at least you have a plan. The other part of this is having the right foods available to you when it is time to eat. The worst thing that can happen (and many fall into this trap) is when you finally do get hungry, you start to scramble just to find something to eat that's decent just to kill the hunger. That's not the right way to eat. If you know that you may not have access to the right food each day, it is your responsibility to have your meals prepared in advance so that when it's time to eat at your allotted time, you can just grab, heat up and eat. For me personally, I like to use Sundays as my prep day. I'll cook some lunches and dinners for the beginning of the week and separate them in Tupperware. During times when I don't cook, due to time constraints, I will outsource this and hire a company that cooks and delivers healthy prepared meals. There are many out there you can use that taste great. Just make sure you are aware of the ingredients they use and how they cook everything. Breakfast is easy for me. Every morning I spend about five to ten minutes scrambling some eggs that I put in Tupperware to bring to work with me. It's important to make this step in your stress free diet a priority but stress free. Remember the saying, "failing to plan is planning to fail."

The NEW Food Pyramid

Carbohydrates:

Fruit - Berries, Apple, Grapefruit, Pears, Oranges

Starches & Grains - Sweet Potatoes, Brown Rice, Quinoa, Wheat Berries, Brown Rice Pasta

Cereals - Oats, Ezekiel (Brand Only)

GOOD FATS:

Oil - Flaxseed oil, Olive Oil, Peanut Oil, Coconut Oil, Palm Oil, From Nuts and Whole Soybeans

Solids - Eggs, Avocados, Almonds, Walnuts and Pecans

Some animal fat

Protein and Vegetables:

Dairy – Eggs, Yogurt, Cheese, Milk (Almond Milk if Lactose-Free)

Meat – Lean Chicken, Lean Beef, Lean Turkey

Fish – Salmon, Tilapia, Orange Ruffy, Flounder, Tuna, Bass, Snapper, Filet of Sole, Halibut

Vegetables - Broccoli, Cabbage, Brussels Sprouts, Asparagus, Cauliflower, Spinach, Mushrooms, Kale

** *Cruciferous vegetables- Arugula, Bok choy, Broccoli, Brussels sprouts, Cabbage, Cauliflower, Collard greens, Horseradish, Kale, Radishes, Rutabaga, Turnips, Watercress, Wasabi*mon

SAMPLE STRESS FREE DIET AROUND WORK-OUT SCHEDULE

Like I said earlier, the key to a stress free diet designed to make you leaner is knowing when to eat your meals and what combination of foods. In the following sample, what I have done is scheduled a moderate carbohydrate day only on the days you workout more intense (ex: strength training days), assuming you train three days per week. The days you do not workout or workout less intensely, are the days in which your carbohydrate intake will be reduced and your healthy fat intake increased. This is designed specifically to give you the energy and nutrients required but at the same time lose body fat. For this plan, we use Saturday as our cheat meal day, followed by a detox day on Sunday.

MONDAY, WEDNESDAY, AND FRIDAY OR HEAVY WORK OUT DAYS:
(LIGHT CARB DAYS)

Breakfast: 3 whole eggs scrambled
Snack or post workout: Protein shake with fresh fruit and low fat or skim milk and water
Lunch: Healthy salad with lean meat/protein and vegetables
Snack: Salads topped with lean meats/protein (tomatoes, handful of nuts, ¼ avocado, onions, vegetables, etc.)
Dinner: Wild rice or sweet potato with grilled chicken and balsamic vinegar and olive oil as dressing.

*At night drink chamomile tea with lemon

TUESDAY AND THURSDAY OR NON-WORKOUT DAYS: (HIGH PROTEIN AND FAT/NO CARB)

Late Breakfast: Hard boiled whole eggs (3)
Lunch: Salads topped with lean meats/protein (tomatoes, handful of nuts, ¼ avocado, onions, vegetables, etc.)
Snack: Almonds (unsalted) or Walnuts (unsalted)
Dinner: Teriyaki Salmon or Steamed/baked/grilled/boiled fish and vegetables

*Friday night (optional) 1 glass of wine

SATURDAY- CHEAT DAY!

Breakfast: 2-3 eggs scrambled. 1 piece of fruit
Lunch: Healthy salad with grilled chicken and balsamic vinegar and olive oil as dressing
Dinner: Have whatever you want within reason
* 2 Drinks (optional)

SUNDAY- FAST

2-3 Detox drinks during the day:
- Kale
- Pineapple chunks
- Half banana
- Scoop of wheat germ (Optional)

- Blueberries
- Water

Dinner: Family dinner- Lean steak and sweet potato with veggies. *No drinks

HERE IS A LIST OF SPICES YOU CAN USE DURING A WEIGHT LOSS PHASE:

Mrs. Dash
Black Pepper
Crushed Red Pepper
Garlic
Garlic powder
Parsley
Oregano
Basil
Turmeric

DON'T COUNT CALORIES EVER AGAIN

I get this question all the time. How many calories should I be taking in daily? Before I answer that question, let's define what a calorie is. The calorie is a metric unit of energy or commonly called a unit of food energy. So in order for our bodies to function each day we have a certain requirement of calories needed for energy output. Let's talk about where we get those calories. All of the calories from our food are divided into proteins, fats and carbohydrates. How many calories are in a gram of each?

1 gram of protein	= 4 calories
1 gram of fat	= 6 calories
1 gram of carbohydrate	= 4 calories

What does this tell you right off the bat? A diet high in fats will contain a lot of calories, right? Does this mean you can automatically eat a low fat diet and lose weight? No! It doesn't really work that way. Now it is said that in order to lose weight you should take in less calories than you expend. This is true to some extent, but it is not a very clear statement and that is what I hope to clarify. First, you need to ask yourself how much weight you really need to lose compared to if you just need to tone up and lose some excess body fat. If you are currently considered obese, focusing on generally lowering your caloric intake is probably a good idea. If toning up and losing body fat percentage is your goal, then focusing on calories is probably not the best plan and can become complicated. Let me explain further. Before you even worry about calories you need to pay attention to the quality of the calories. Many of the weight loss products and systems out there spend a lot of time on calorie counting and point system, which allow the person to eat empty calories. Again, I'm going to stress that the quality of the calorie is more important than how many. A diet that is evenly balanced and full of clean whole foods will end up working out to be lower in calories in the long run. Even if you're eating 5-6 meals a day, if you are eating clean, well-balanced meals, your total caloric intake will be at a suitable amount. The problem arises when people restrict their calories way too much in hopes of losing weight. What this ultimately does is waste away the tissue in our bodies, which drives our metabolism. This tissue is known as "muscle". I'm always telling my inner circle coaching clients to feed your muscles, not your stomach. Your level of exercise and what types of exercise you do will also determine how many calories you need. Even though you might be watching your calorie intake, your exercise expendure plays a major role. If you are eating fairly low calories, then maybe you just need to step up your training.

HABITS

The best thing you can do to improve your habits (besides following the brain detox properties and the six key motivators) is to limit the choices available to you. One of the biggest problems we face today is that we have too many choices. Everything is at our fingertips and easily accessible, which is causing our brains to be less focused and dialed into what we need to be. We're finding this to be time with regard to things like food choices, spouses, and relationships. It's time to start simplifying your life. Our ancestors were limited on their choices and lived much simpler. I'm not saying that we have to go back to medieval times, but we can keep it simple and consistent. Don't just add good habits, replace bad habits with the good ones. What are you willing to give up? Your level of acceptable behavior must change. A great book to read on the power of small habits is "The Compound Effect" by Darren Hardy.

The most important habit I impress upon my coaching clients is to change their morning ritual. This by far sets the tone for the rest of your day and will create a better momentum for the rest of the day. It all starts with your daily actions, which will eventually lead to what you really want out of yourself and life. If you don't start your day off right from the moment you wake up, then the rest of the day will become more of a challenge. Next thing you know, you've wasted another day which could have been used to move you closer to your goals. What does your morning ritual look like right now? Is it in line with your goals in life or in health and fitness? Or are you rushing just to get out the door to start your hectic day. Maybe you just have time for a quick cup of coffee and throw on the news to see the weather or hear about who got shot in the projects, or watch some silly news personality doing a skit. You then rush the kids out of the house so they get to school on time. So what happens to you? You're rushed, a little stressed and eventually you get hungry a few hours later and end up reaching for the muffins and donuts at the office. Your morning ritual is what sets the tone for a productive day to improve you both physically and mentally. The morning is actually the perfect time to set you up for success each and every day. But you have to change your morning ritual!

Let's take a look at a morning ritual that will set you up for success both physically and mentally. If time is a problem, get yourself to bed an hour earlier and then wake up an hour earlier to give you more time. This might be a little challenging at first, but you will adjust to it. Besides, with a better morning ritual you will begin to wake up with more energy and vigor. Next is what you eat. Now I know many of you will tell me, "Greg I'm just not hungry or feel like making anything." Well my answer to that is starting to train you little by little to eat. Now is the best time to start your metabolism working. It will also help ward off those late night hunger snacks. The morning is a great time to start your day by feeding your mind something positive. Turn off the news (because you are not missing anything, trust me!) Spend a few minutes reading, meditating, breathing, or brainstorming. This will probably be your one moment of peace before the day starts. Sometimes you don't have control on how the day goes, but you can control how it starts and finishes. Make a list of things to accomplish and get done for the day. Preparation = less worry = less stress = SUCCESS.

GREG'S PIA'S (Put Into Action)

- Get important supplements. I like to order them online. Email my assistant at support@thebraindetoxdiet.com and she will give you our recommended sources for quality and fair priced supplements.

- Make an eating schedule in your appointment book or phone.

- Go food shopping for only the whole foods you need to prepare meals and snacks.

- Prepare a few meals and snacks in Tupperware and zip lock bags for a few days at a time.

- Don't stress over calories.

- Eat very clean and structured during the week.

- Give yourself a good progress month to kick start your new body.

- If you have a long way to go, don't get overwhelmed. Replace one habit at a time.

- Feed your muscles, not your stomach.

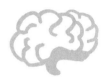

Chapter 8

GAIN MOMENTUM

Think Big/ Start small. That's my motto. The reason why most people fail or never get started on anything is because they get too overwhelmed!

You have to start small. Whenever you want to get started on a new venture like starting a new diet and setting goals, you should start small. I know you have big goals and aspirations and that's great, you should! But trying to accomplish those goals can be an overwhelming experience. That's why starting somewhere small and working your way up your success ladder is the way to go.

Let's say your main goal is that you want to get back in shape. Instead of getting overwhelmed with having to workout everyday and totally change your diet by eating perfectly, you could take this approach: Start with a three day a week structured workout routine and just replace certain meals with healthy, quality food. You can even add a healthy snack in between one of your meals or even just improve your breakfast.

For me, starting and owning a business was something I always wanted. Becoming a gym owner seemed like a daunting task, so I started small. First, I became a free-lance trainer and paid rent at another guy's gym with just a few clients. Next, I hired another trainer and filed their schedule. (And then another!) Eventually I moved into a starter studio for a few years, which eventually led to the gym, I own now which was my ultimate goal!

I started small and little by little hit each goal. I didn't get too overwhelmed. Are you ready to start knocking off your small goals to eventually reach the big ones? Give yourself a very short-term goal. Prepare for that goal and see it through. Once you hit your first short term goal, which was easily achievable, enjoy and identify with the result. This will begin a momentum, which will allow your focus to build stronger and stronger.

There is a study done by two psychotherapists who spent a year interviewing and compiling data from the happiest people they could find in 33 different countries. Their research found that an individual's level of happiness is determined largely by one four-letter word. What's your guess? Most will say LOVE. Some will say CASH. What the therapists found was interesting. It is nothing that occurs outside ourselves. This four-letter word was RISK. Love, cash and joy come to those who RISK.

Remember, you are no longer the old you. The old you would give up by now. The old you would let a few days of no results discourage you. The old you would let one slip up derail you from your ultimate goal. The old you would tell yourself, "well I tried". The old you will say I can try again next month. The old you is gone! That mindset has died with the old you. This is the NEW YOU! The more EMPOWERED YOU. The you that is in control of your destiny. Your destiny is to look in the mirror knowing that you accomplished greatness and have taken control of your health and look your best!

Now is the time. You don't get second chances at greatness! You are at that pivotal moment where you can accomplish this. Don't give up right before the finish line. I believe in all of you! I want you ALL to succeed. Don't let me want you to succeed more than YOU!

The best question you can ask yourself is: "If we were meeting 1 year from today and you were to look back over that year, what has to happen during that year for you to feel happy about your progress?" From there I would like you to write down three areas in your life that need improvement and three obstacles you need to overcome. Now circle the top priority goals in both categories. Now that you have your vision, you can also be aware of your biggest improvement area and obstacles to overcome. Change both of these and you will get closer to that vision.

I failed at a lot of things.

- I set a goal of having 100 family members at my gym in the first year of opening my gym. I ended up with 92 members after the first year. **= Fail**
- I set a goal of making 200 people a part of my gym family after our expansion within the first six months. We had 175. **= Fail**

- One summer I wanted to go from 15% body fat down to 7%. By summer I was at 9%. **= Fail**
- I set a goal to compete and place top 3 overall in a warrior challenge one summer. I didn't place top 3 overall, I just finished the challenge and was top 10 in one event. **= Fail**

Now you can look at each of these as failures, but I would call it PROGRESS. If I didn't set high goals and standards for myself then I would never have helped 92 people in one year feel better and achieve more. I wouldn't have 175 beautiful people kicking butt and lifting each other to be better in the first six months of expanding. I also wouldn't have changed my body and gotten down to 9% body fat that summer. I wouldn't have competed and completed an extremely tough warrior challenge.

Don't sell yourself short if you are not exactly where you want to be and DO NOT start feeling like a failure. If you set the bar high, those failures become PROGRESS and you achieve more than you would if you didn't set the bar high. Do not get caught up with your perceived limitations. Think big and start small to attain those goals. As you step up the ladder of progress, you will just about find that the impossible has just become a little bit more possible.

It's your time right now to rise above your current state and become a better version of yourself. Use this new inner focus and energy to strengthen yourself. No more procrastinating on what you want from life, on your dreams and no more just getting through the day. You are better than that! Make your contribution to the universe by raising your frequency and making the most of your short time in that body. Time is running out. Use everyday to your advantage. Stop waiting for the perfect time because you will only be followed by disappointment.

Take action right now! I have just given you a plan to follow. Take chances, be persistent and don't live in fear. Go beyond where you are. There's always a way. As you read my last words to you, know that from today going forward you are already a more complete person. Today is the first day of the rest of your life. Go create your life and live your dreams right now.

"REACH FOR THE STARS AND HIT THE MOON"

GREG'S PIA'S (PUT INTO ACTION)

- Don't wait for perfect. Start now!

- Start small. Start by changing one thing at a time.

- Write down your goals. Pen to paper is powerful. Write one big crazy goal and then monthly mini goals.

- Don't let anyone stop you from achieving your goals. You're in control of your own life.

- Failing is just falling short of goals. So fail forward and fail a lot. Every time you do, you get closer to your dreams.

Happiness = Stop focusing on the things you can't change and start focusing on the things you CAN change.

LIVE LIKE A CHAMPION:

Face your fears.
Champions of life have fears, they just face them.

Speak up when you believe something is wrong.
Champions will fight for the greater good.

Don't complain.
Champions of life don't complain, they work through it.

Don't hold back your love.
Champions love hard even when at risk.

Think before you react.
Champions do not let their emotions get the best of them.

Don't do anything mediocre.
Champions give their best in everything they do. You know what your best is.

Do things for people, but expect nothing in return...ever.
Champions don't keep score.

Have balance in your life.
Champions make time for family, career, spirituality and their health.

When things get hard, fight through it and don't quit.
Champions give it 100% to the end and then fight for more.

Always look to evolve and embrace change.
Champions always look to improve and thrive under adversity.

Take the bad that has happened in your life and channel that into doing something great for yourself.
Champions use past experiences as the fuel to ignite a burning desire to succeed.

Pay attention to your input and protect yourself from who and what you listen to.
Champions fill their sub-conscious minds with positive life enhancing reinforcement.

Be more ruthless with time management.
Champions don't waste time on nonsense but instead use their time efficiently.

Do not depend on anyone else but yourself.
Champions take control of their own lives and get the job done.

Don't just try to get by.
Champions live with purpose and passion.

Don't look at this list and say, "easier said than done!"
Champions do not look for excuses!

-Greg Crawford

BIBLIOGRAPHY:

"Man's Search for Meaning" by Viktor Frankl

"Silent power" by Stewart Wilde

"E Squared" by Pam Grout

"The power of your subconscious mind" by Joseph Murphy

"Nutrition and physical degeneration" by Weston A. Price

The antioxidant miracle" by Lester Packer and Carol Colman

"The super antioxidants" by James Balch

"The One thing" by Gary Keller and Jay Papasan

"The compound effect" by Darren Hardy

"Awaken the giant within" by Anthony Robbins

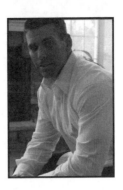

ABOUT AUTHOR

Greg Crawford is a long time fitness and nutrition expert and entrepreneur who is one of the leaders in his industry. After starting his own gym and further expanding his business, Greg has helped hundreds of people transform not only their bodies but their lives as well. After creating his popular and successful 30 day weight loss detox challenge, Greg started applying the Brain Detox principles with these people which helped them make lasting changes in their lives. From the request of many, Greg published his principles and philosophies along with his own personal story in *The Brain Detox Diet* (*www.TheBrainDetoxDiet.com*).

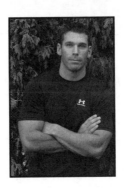

GREG'S PROGRAMS:

Would You Like To Have Me In Your Corner To Personally Coach You and Set You Up With A Fitness and Life Game Plan? I Want To Be Your Personal Life Coach.

Dear Friend,

I'm looking for "dream" clients that I can make massive life changes with. If that's you, I will personally work with you one-on-one in your life to help you feel awesome, look awesome and reflect awesome to the world.

The first thing I'm going to do for you is to personally help you create a strategic plan to jump start you into success.

For only $200 we'll have a face-to-face Skype phone call for about 30-45 minutes.

(After doing this almost 15 years straight, I've gotten pretty good at fast results).

During this call, I will break down the WHAT, WHY and HOW.

- WHAT exactly you want out of your fitness and life goals
- What your "WHY" is. This is where we share and get to the core of your motivation.
- HOW we will achieve this together as a team. This is where I set you up with a game plan.

At the end of this initial planning session you will have more clarity and a direction with what to do next.

It really is that simple.

WARNING - TIME IS A FACTOR

This opportunity is extremely limited because of the intense one-on-one time needed in order to provide you with results. Therefore, it is physically impossible for me to work with more than a handful of people.

Schedule a strategy call with Greg. Let me design and help you with a life and fitness game plan. You need a coach like me in your corner. After reading my book, I want to help you put it into action and begin your new journey.

Email support@thebraindetoxdiet.com to schedule your Skype call with Greg.

You'll also learn about Greg's ongoing coaching programs.

SPEAKING:

Have me speak at your event or organization. The Brain Detox Workshop will help you be:

- A mentally stronger person
- More focused
- Better at blocking stress and negative roadblocks
- Leaner and healthier

WHO IS THIS TALK FOR:

- Corporations
- Weight loss groups
- Fundraisers

Speaking fee: $1000 plus travel.

*(Speaking fee can be waived with purchasing a copy of Greg's book for each attendee.)

To schedule Greg or for further information:

Email at **support@thebraindetoxdiet.com**